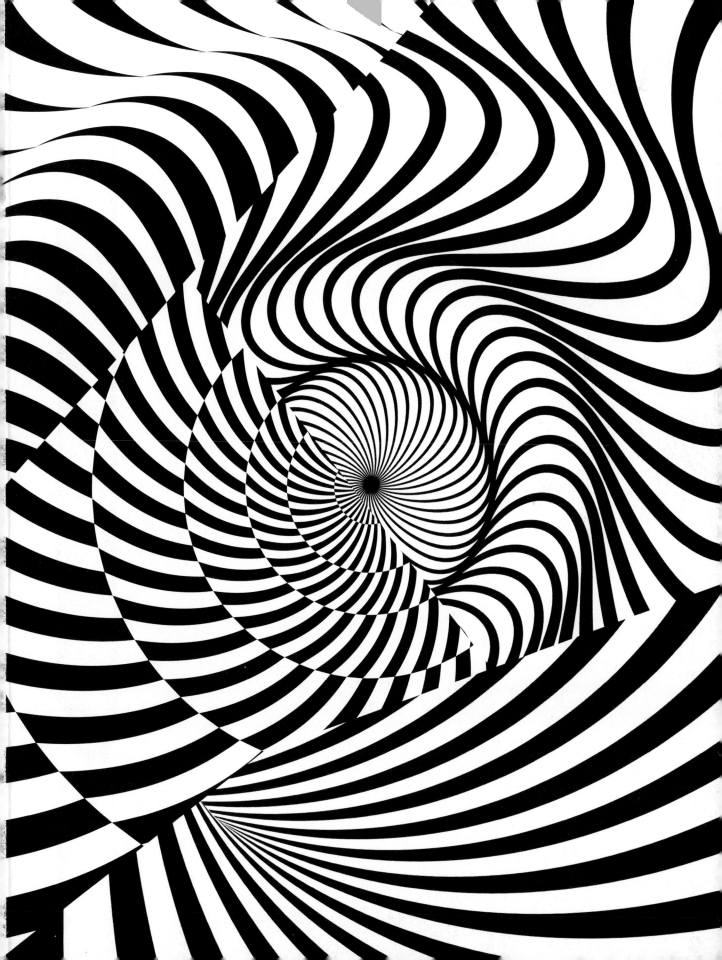

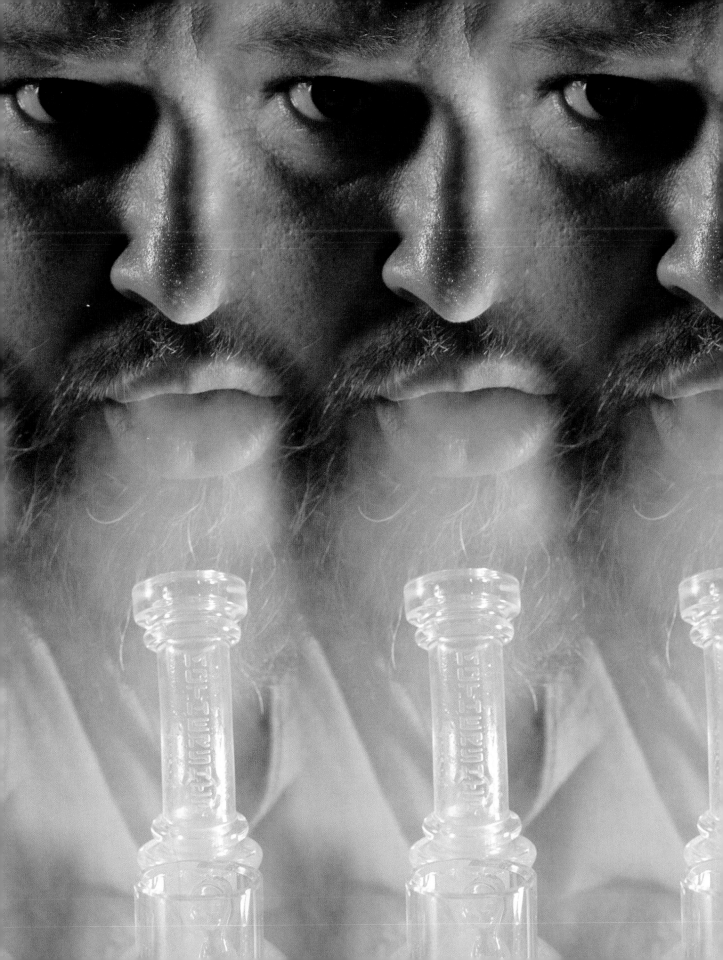

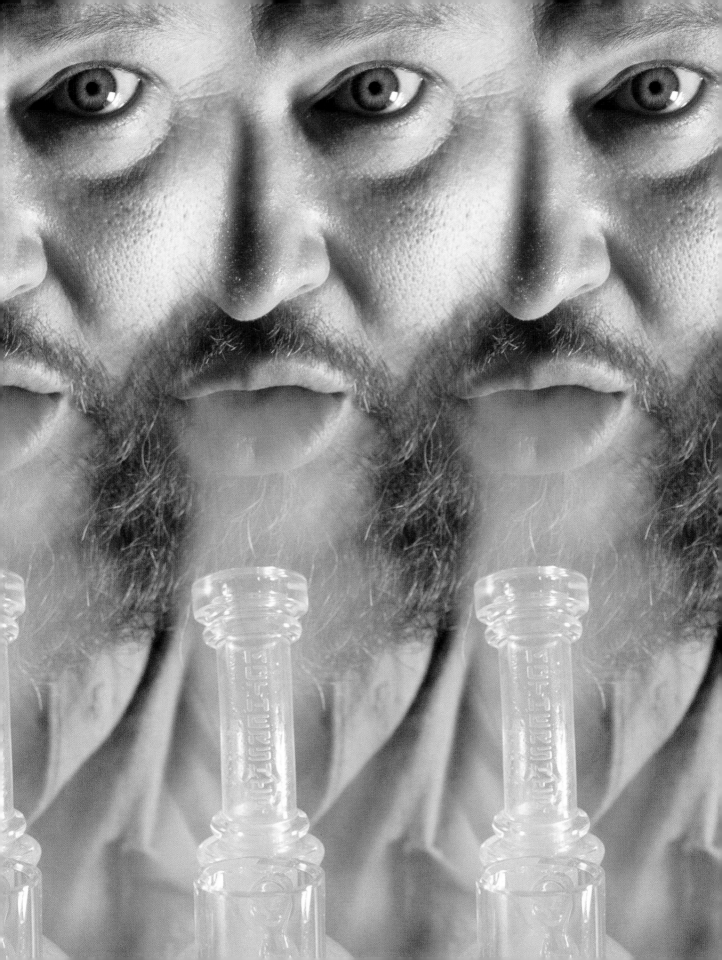

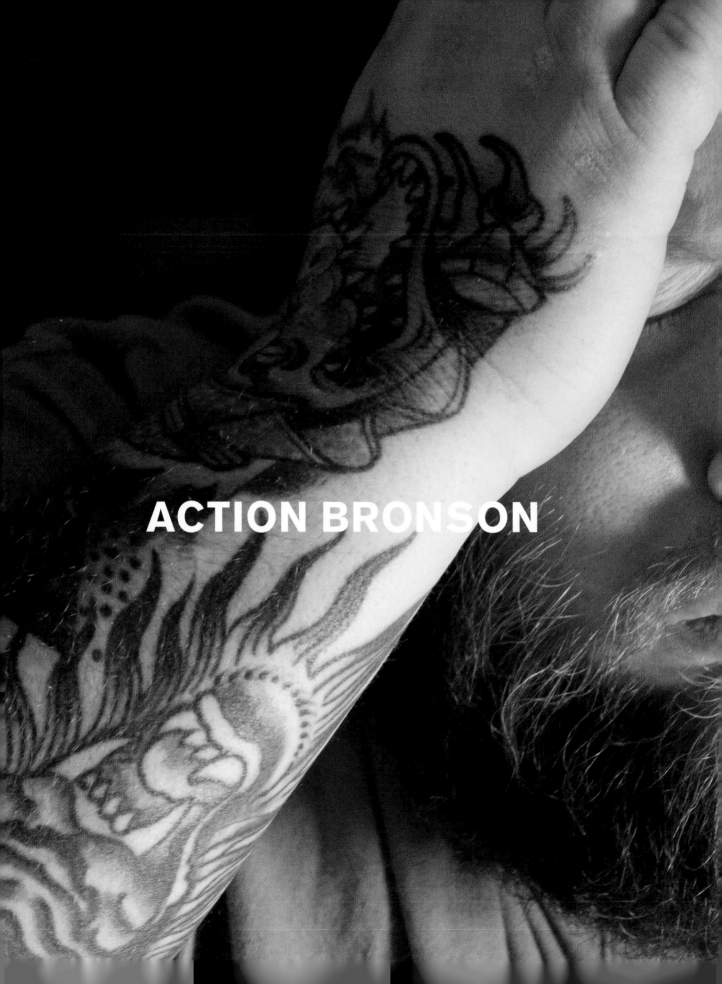

ACTION BRONSON

STONED BEYOND BELIEF

with Rachel Wharton

Abrams Image, New York

Introduction

*THIS BOOK HAS BEEN A BURDEN
TO WRITE.
THIS HASN'T BEEN AN EASY BOOK
TO WRITE.*

IT'S TAKING AWAY FROM MY HIGH TIME.

MY THEM TIME.

MY ME TIME.

*BUT THIS BOOK IS A BIG DEAL,
BECAUSE WEED CHANGED MY LIFE.*

I think that weed was the best influence on me, period, all the time, starting with the path it has taken me on. It changed the course of mad things in my life. As a youth, pre-weed, I was playing football, I was doing good in school, I was in shape. I'm not blaming the weed for what changed, just that I liked weed so much, I decided to give everything else up and go chase my dreams. My real dreams: smoking weed every day.

My priorities were a lot different back then. Smoking weed wasn't like a ritual for me early on. I didn't realize how spiritual it was to me until later on. Now smoking it, preparing to smoke it, that is my therapy. Weed is my companion: I always have my tree with me. If I'm up on a fucking mountaintop, it's going to be me and tree. The tree of life, you know. And I smoke weed wherever I am because it is who I am. I feel like you should always be who you are—why try to hide something? I can't hide anything, that's how I am: I am just myself to the extreme.

Plus, weed helps me get through the trauma.

Weed does so many things. Weed should be a superhero.

Weed can expand your horizons: You don't think the same way you used to think. That's what drew me to it, the chance to have that altered state of reality. Because sometimes you don't want to be in your reality, so you're trying to get yourself as much as you can into another one, and then that just becomes your norm. But it's an enjoyable norm: It's not like a medically induced lithium norm. In fact, my awareness is on the craziest peak ever– self-awareness, nature awareness. My self-discovery is off the charts.

A lot of people who are depressed or have anxiety, they don't need to go to a shrink, they just need to smoke some weed. I really do feel that way. A lot of great people found themselves through weed. Everyone who likes great food and is not a stuck-up piece of garbage smokes weed. Or has done something similar. Outside-the-box thinkers smoke weed.

Weed puts you on another plane; it is a conduit for happiness, for knowledge seeking, for understanding, and also for release and total relaxation and comfortability. It doesn't matter where you are: When you're stoned, you're your own world, and that's all that matters to you.

Weed just puts you in a space of good

vibes and good celestial feelings and good celestial energies. Way back in the day all we could buy were nickel bags, and we used to call smoking them "nick at night." We'd work all day, and at the end of the day we'd look at each other and say, Nick at Night? And we'd all agree, and we'd go back to my friend's house, smoke on his little balcony in his room, and we'd be cracking up and just enjoying our lives.

People like getting high; it feels good. It just really feels incredible.

Weed is also a connector. Man, I've been far and wide in this country and this world, and weed has let me meet so many people. People all over the world often stop me in the street to try to smoke with me: If they don't know English, they just stop you with a smoke in their hand. They'll start with where they're from. *Maroc. Maroc.* Then they'll say *hashish, hashish,* and then they'll say the name of their favorite football player, usually some famous French footballer–it's ridiculous, but it works. I know what they're saying: Let's smoke some weed.

Somebody says, *Yo, I got some great fucking weed.* Aiight, I go. I call their bluff.

Because I love weed. I do. I need it every day. I diagnosed myself with extreme ADHD–all the letters you could possibly have–and this is the only thing that slows all that down. I can't sit still, I can't stand still, I can't stop shaking my leg. I've been fidgety since grade school. I feel like I need the weed to combat my hyperactivity. So it's medicine.

It's also food and drink. It's cereal. It's fucking steak. I could be as hungry as a motherfucker right now and be dreaming of a steak. If I smoke a joint, it's just as good. I'm eventually going to want that steak a million times more, but in that moment I'm smoking, I'll be satisfied.

I get Stoned Beyond Belief every single day of my life. But as you smoke and you smoke and you smoke, you build up a tolerance, and you're constantly searching for that old high school stoned. That's what I'm looking for: your eyes really low, tearing up, almost shut, a big grin on your face, hungry as a motherfucker, eating chips, the chips falling all over you, ashes on your shirt, just acting really silly. You're like the old cars with the pop-up headlights, where one of them is stuck halfway down. You want to feel like you lost your phone: Where's my phone? It's literally right next to you.

That's the high I am trying to find, that weed that's going to get me high like it did back then. That's Stoned Beyond Belief. I'm still fucking searching for that. I seek that feeling every day.

Introduction

1.

THE WEST COAST

There's so much amazing stuff going on in America right now with weed, and it's mainly on the West Coast. Nearly everything I know that's fire comes from Out West. First, weed is legal there, so all the amazing botanists and growers and artisanal hash makers moved out that way. There's so many good people involved in the cannabis community and culture out there, every kind of product is made, every kind of byproduct or tool. You'll visit and come back with all kinds of elixirs and tinctures, pens and oils and products. Weed cream that doesn't get you high but will cure your back pain or your eczema. And now the West Coast has opened the doors for all of us. Their knowledge has expanded to Colorado and Michigan and Maine and Massachusetts and the world.

For me, a lot of my own weed transformation came in LA a few years ago. I became awoken to the weed universe, to the bounty and beauty that the land provides. LA was where I first got turned on to really good weed, and then to extracts and oil and next-level hash: Right now there is no place like the Pacific Northwest for hash and the good strains of weed and just the fire. And Colorado? It's all there too. So many who grow weed or make weed products are fans of music in general, and they love to offer their thanks to me for making music by allowing me to taste the best flavors of weed in the world. Over the years it's become a beautiful, harmonious relationship among grower, maker, and connoisseur.

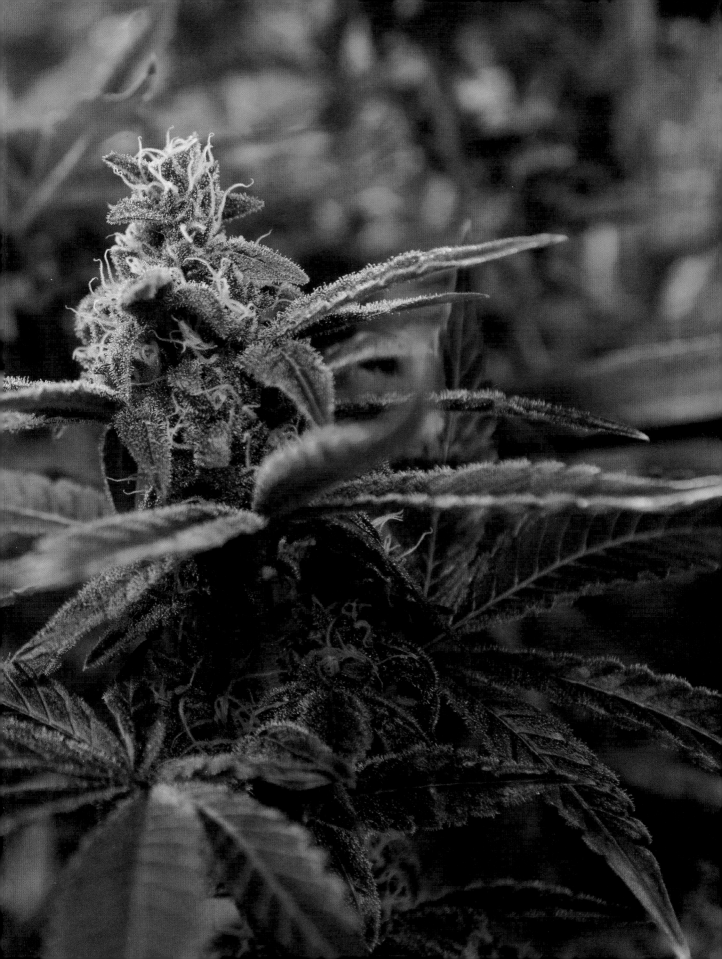

A Conversation with The Alchemist, LA-bred, About the History of West Coast Weed

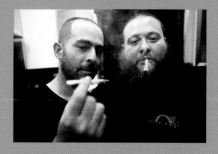

AB: I gotta get more poignant about this. Al, do you have any input here? You don't have any input, do you wanna lay down?

AL: 'Bout what?

AB: One hundred things weed-related is what I'm trying to get at. But there's so many things. Do you have any things from your past? Can we interview you? We can do What Al Likes.

AL: We can talk about weed, mannnnn. I have a different perspective.

AB: I know you do; this is why I want to get your perspective.

AL: 'Course it's different. We all came up different. Smoking different. I grew up in LA, where the weed was. The good weed, if it ended up here, it usually came from the West Coast, where it was more plentiful.

AB: You're right.

AL: I think the people you knew were more the dealers. And I knew a lot of growers, 'cause I knew hippies and dudes growing up; it was the hippie thing. You had to know somebody, like, exclusivity, it was a different thing. It's hard to explain now for the kids.

AB: So tell me what you mean, like only the ill people had the ill shit?

AL: It was impossible to get certain types of weed, because it was from just one person. You had to know one guy, who knew another guy, who knew this weirdo—it's like in the Cheech and Chong movies.

AB: Yeah, yeah, yeah, yeah.

AL: It was, like, more quiet and secretive, and even then there was only little bits of it, so it's not like it is now.

AB: Where we're running around with fucking huge bags.

AL: There was no steady flow of good weed, so it was, like, to have a connection or to know someone was the only way to have good weed back then. It was, like, fucking special, like something you didn't really share with a lot of people, because you couldn't then. Only a little bit would be grown, and then it would be bullshit for weeks. And like now, the sour—it's always around, it never goes away. Never.

AB: At one time over here I only knew dealers; it was all coming from Canada.

AL: But that's still probably West Coast weed.

AB: They would always call it BC, they would call it Beasters. You know, it was this big, chunky, disgusting weed that just had no flavor, it was just this hard-core bullshit, you know? Beaster weed, it was the most common weed at the time, it was kind of like regs.

AL: They would call it BC, for British Columbia, 'cause it was Canadian. It looked like trees. You know those toy train sets, you know the little trees? It looked like stiff little perfectly shaped little trees. It was like mass-produced bullshit. I knew about it—we had that out there too. But it's always been different, because East Coast is more business based, because the culture of weed and growing it is on the West Coast. Somebody else might say that we're trippin', 'cause they grew up out here in the nineties and were growing weed, but to my knowledge, from my perspective, the good weed always came from the West Coast.

AB: Always. I mean, once I started learning about good weed, it was always from the West.

AL: 'Cause that's where the culture was, and the hippies.

AB: That's where the know-how was, that's where the knowledge was.

AL: It was also the climate—even OG, the original OG, was supposedly ocean grown. It was supposed to be a strain that was from Santa Cruz. Ocean grown, that's the OG. We can look it up: There's, like, myths—some people say it exists naturally. It was grown outdoors, by the ocean, in Santa Cruz.

AB: Oh, shit. A lot of weird things grow near water, like near ocean. Remember when we were in fucking Australia? All those crazy things? All those crazy algaes and crazy shit that grew right there, all those little sea plants. A lot of things that are near the ocean are flavored by the ocean. When I was in Croatia, they were telling us that the lambs were better-tasting lamb because they graze near the ocean, and they get salted by the sea, by the mist from the sea. They're literally living their lives being seasoned every day. How crazy is that, they're being brined every day?

AL: When I moved here in '95, '96 and I was in college, none of the roommates I had had any idea of the shit that I had—that shit was foreign to them. They had never seen it before, they were like, what is this? Chronic? It's changed so much now. It's changed in so many ways. Fuck, man, there's so many levels in how it's changed, but definitely the taboo side of it has changed. That opens up the door for so much shit, you know.

AB: Everyone smokes now, it's like a thing to do.

AL: I think what stopped it when we were kids was that they equaled it to, like, cocaine, drugs. It was still bad in the eighties. Bad. But now, my brother's kids, they have a different view on weed than I did, it's not being pushed as such a bad thing. It's not being endorsed for kids, but it's not like cocaine or fucking pills.

AB: I mean Snoop Dogg. They see Snoop Dogg—he's cool, he's smoking weed.

AL: For people like us who have been smoking weed our whole lives, the fact that it's becoming legal now isn't groundbreaking for us. I mean, it is groundbreaking, but it opens up a whole new door for the grandmother and the parent who never smoked weed their whole life, 'cause it was wrong, taboo, and culturally incorrect. Now it's like drinking wine, and they're going to start smoking weed in their sixties, and they're going to love it, and that's going to open a whole 'nother market for older people just getting introduced to it.

AB: And for the edible game, because there's so much more, and pens and this and that.

AL: There's all these people who never did it their whole lives, and for whatever reasons, and they're going to realize this is great and doesn't hurt you, and that's a whole new market.

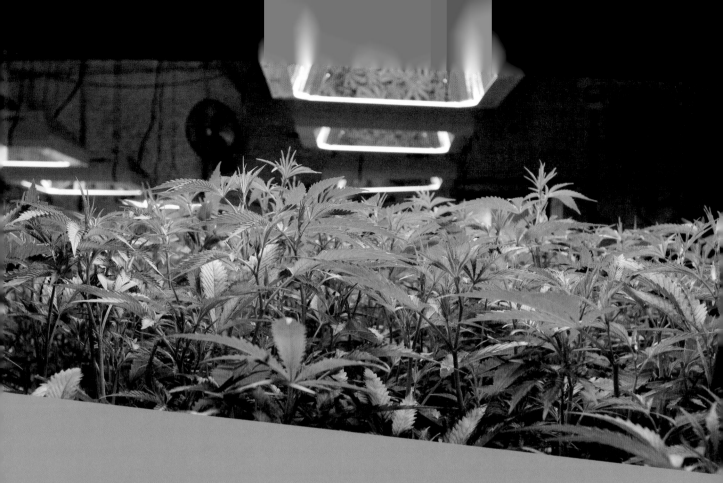

AB: We were already in. It had me at hello.

AB: I want the foreword to this book to be written by weed. See, that's a high-ass thought. Yo, I want weed to write the book, yo. It'd be crazy, if it was, like, from the perspective of weed . . . cough, cough. . . . Weed has opened so many doors for me in my life and made me so many friends. If you don't have any friends, smoke weed, and you'll have friends, trust me. I didn't have any friends until I started smoking weed. I'm joshing you. No, but it solidifies relationships.

AL: Weed will get you through times of no money better than money will get you through times of no weed.

AB: Spoken like a poet.

AL: No, man, that's an expression. I've heard that one before. You know that one, that's so true.

AB: So true.

AL: You got all the money, and you can't get no weed.

AB: I don't give a shit about the money. Give me my damn weed now.

AL: Word up, what am I going to do with all this money?

AB: I'm not high.

AL: There's, like, two different sides to this thing: There's the stoner fucking idiot eating pizza and playing video games, and there's, like, the spiritual fucking guy who tries to balance his fucking chi or whatever. Weed is different for different people.

AB: The cancer patient.

AL: There's so many different levels of this.

AB: The father trying to bond with the kid. The mother trying to bond with the kid—you never know, man. Desperate times call for desperate measures.

AL: It's clearly a gift. Weed.

AB: It's a gift from the heavens.

AL: From nature, in general. C'mon, there are a million plants, all across the world, you know what I am saying.

AB: That's what I'm saying. I think it's very similar to fruit, a gift.

AL: And not trying to get really stoney, 'cause this is what you get around those stoners, and they go down this path, but you wanna talk about all the uses for hemp? You really want to go down that path, right now? Yo, real talk, though, one time motherfuckers were putting me on, like a real stoner guy, and he was like, basically, you can change the whole world with hemp. That shit is biodegradable. You can use it for gas—it can be gasoline, it can replace plastic, plastic never biodegrades, but they said hemp can replace plastic and it goes back to the earth. Once you get into that shit, there's probably a lot of reasons why it's not legal, 'cause it's, like, big business, you know what I mean? The plastic, the fucking fuel business? And he was serious.

AB: [pretending to be a real stoner guy] Yo, it can replace plastic, dog.

AL: You know that line.

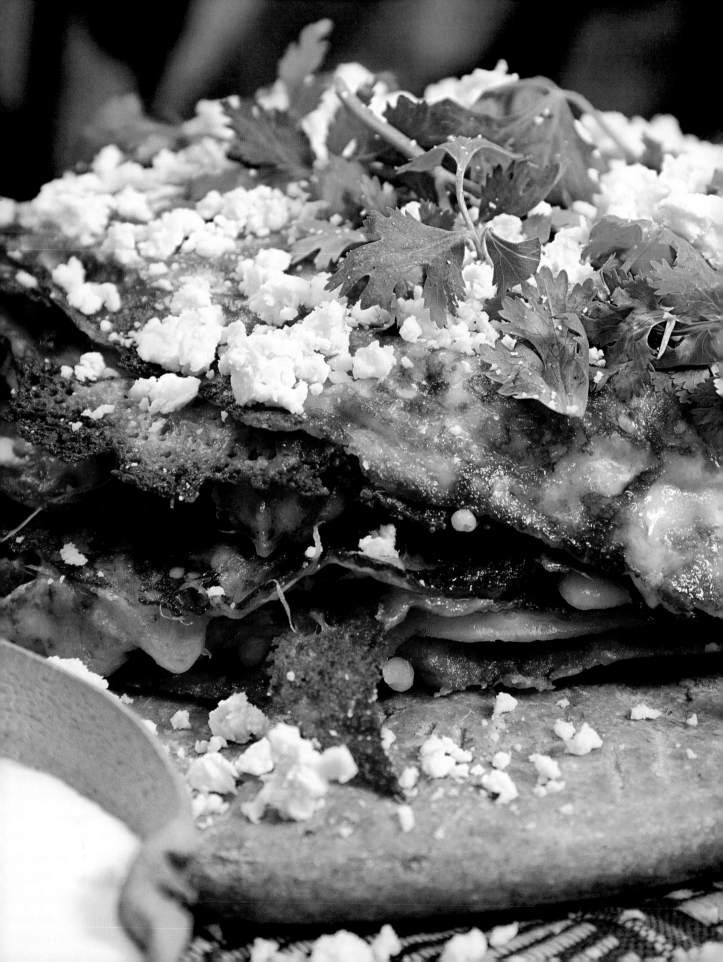

This is the ultimate stoner food, 100 percent—it takes ten minutes, and you can have all this in the fridge all the time. I've made this many nights, many a night. So much so that I've perfected my recipe. They always suck at restaurants, but at home they can be amazing. You want a lot of cheese, because you want it to ooze out and get crispy so it looks like a sun. But you make a mound in the middle so it doesn't come out too fast. Sometimes with a quesadilla you have no cheese in the middle—this way, that's not going to happen. And you want mixed cheeses, because that crispy edge with cheeses mixed is next. Then you want a little spice, to wake you up, plus a little vinegar from the hot sauce, that brings everything together. You don't even need to dip it in anything—it's already seasoned. Sure, it's a fucking quesadilla, but when you can make it yourself, it's so satisfying, it's like you've accomplished something.

Makes 1

2 10-inch (25-cm) flour tortillas
¼ cup (60 ml) grated mozzarella cheese
¼ cup (60 ml) grated Cheddar cheese
Melinda's Original Habanero Hot Sauce, or hot sauce of your choosing, to taste
2 tablespoons thinly sliced jalapeño chile, fresh or pickled

1. Heat a skillet over medium-high heat. (I find I don't need oil in the pan to make these, but you could use a little olive oil if you don't believe me.)

2. Place 1 tortilla in the middle of the skillet, then mound both cheeses in the middle of the tortilla, leaving about an inch (2.5 cm) of space around the edge of the tortilla. Sprinkle about 6 splotches of hot sauce all over the cheese, like heavy raindrops. Then place the sliced chiles all over the cheese, tucking them in here and there.

3. Top the quesadilla with the second tortilla. When the cheese has started to melt, press down the center of the quesadilla with a spatula, so the cheese starts to seep out the sides and fry in its own fat. I want you to push the cheese out, to get that rim, that ring of fire.

4. Let the bottom tortilla fully brown, then flip the quesadilla over and let the other tortilla fully brown and the cheese continue to melt and ooze and fry around the edges. You want the cheese to darken and sizzle but not fully burn.

5. When both sides are brown, turn off the heat and put the quesadilla on a cutting board. Let it sit for a second, like a pizza; let the cheese seep back into its situation.

6. Then slice it up—it should crunch, you want to hear it when you cut it. Or you can go crazy, make a bunch of them, stack 'em up, and cut them into wedges like a cake.

2.
Quesadilla
with Crispy

There was a time in my life about a decade ago when all my friends and I would all hang out in–let's call him Frizzante–in Frizzante's basement in Queens. That basement was The Hub for everything: to smoke, to chill, to hang out. You always need a hub, whether it's a hotel room on the road, or Al's house in LA, or the dressing room backstage–the spot where people can come through, to hang, to eat, to play music, to sesh. Now The Hub is my music studio in New York.

But the basement–we always called it The Basement–was the original hub, and the amount of weed that changed hands and that was smoked in that place is unbeliev-able. People would show up from everywhere out of the blue, because you'd always know The Basement was poppin'. There could be thirty people coming through on any given night. My friend's parents hated it, which is why we're not naming any names. We were kicked out many times, though a lot of times we'd just go out, go around the block for ten minutes, then come back. Or we would go to Joey Shift's backyard. I didn't know Joey Shift, but everyone would always talk about him.

It looked like *Wayne's World* down there: couches, subway map, big-screen TV, shitty floor, staircase coming down from the house, a bathroom in the back, and a kitchen, with its own entrance around at the back door. Frizzante even used to rent it to some guy named Arturo, which Frizzante's parents weren't crazy about.

We'd be there all day long, even when my friend wasn't there. Just imagine the craziest hangout possible–smoking, drinking, music, yelling, everything. I watched the Giants win both Super Bowls down there; I watched the Yankees win *multiple World Series* down there.

4.

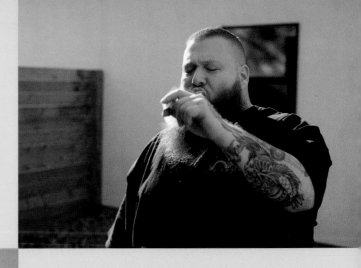

Someone Else's Weed.

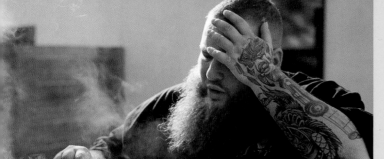

Plus, Scamming and Other Trickery.

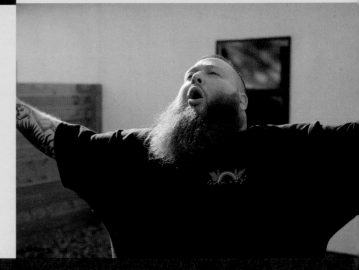

Action Bronson: I sold all the old-school boxing books and autographs my grandfather left me when he died, for weed.

Rachel Wharton: Damn.

Action Bronson: It was always all about weeeeeed.

Rachel Wharton: How much weed did it buy?

Action Bronson: Who knows? Not enough for the tears and hurt I would've caused Irv if he knew

No matter how much weed I have, I'll always tell someone I don't have weed. Always. The thought of them lighting up their weed first sounds so much better than me lighting up my weed first. Of course, this was back in the day: Now I light up all over, left and right, Beverly Hills, fucking Santo Domingo, whatever you want. But for a long time, the thought of not having to pay to get high was the pinnacle of life, like Christmas. Everyone would be, yo, you got weed? and I'd be like, nah. And everyone else would be like, nah. Because everyone lies. Then someone eventually would come up with some weed, and I'd have my weed for later.

Usually, though, you had to make sure to pitch in some money, five here, five there, maybe ten. I always liked to have ten in on the weed for some reason. Fifteen, if I had it. I liked to have a good amount of money on the weed, so I'd get mine. Though luckily there's never really a majority shareholder when you're sharing a blunt: You're not going to tell your boy, yo, you only take one hit, I take two. You just share: Good friends are supposed to share, to get each other drugs, to smoke each other's weed. But not everyone's as generous with their weed, so that's why, when you find that really generous person, you become good friends with them.

I also used to be the king of credit. I had ten dudes on rotation: If I owed this one money for weed, the next one would get the call. Or if one person would take too long to come by, I'd call the next one. Sometimes it would get crossed up, and three mother-fuckers would be coming through at once, like having three girlfriends show up at the same time. Eventually I would pay them: I'd owe people ten, twenty bucks, and I'd be scummy, I'd duck someone one day, paying somebody else their money, fucking the other dude over, a constant circle of credit. I would get the phone call asking for the money, and I would miss that phone call, but when I needed them, I'd call them ten times. (With my StarTAC Motorola, the flip, with the green screen and the antenna that you pulled up with that big plastic piece at the end.) Occasionally, I'd purchase weed straight up, but very occasionally. I

definitely still owe somebody $150 for an ounce. I also remember finagling specific people out of weed: I have the gift of persuasion, and I am charming. Plus, the bottom line if you're a small-time dealer is you either sell the weed or you don't. And I never had an issue with people trying to get me for owing them money: My trickery was on such a small scale, and most people were just dipping their toe into dealing back then.

I would also find creative ways to get money. There could not be a situation where I could be left out in the cold without weed. I've never told anyone this, but I am telling you: When I would work in restaurant kitchens, I would go food shopping at Restaurant Depot. I used to do the purchasing, and I used to skim off the top. So that there would always be money left over, I'd ask for more than I needed, and I wouldn't give back the change. Everybody else knew what I was doing, but I faked reasons to get the cash just for myself, for my own psyche, my own sickness. It was a sickness, and I recognized that there was something wrong with me. But then I would get the rest of the dudes high in the little alley in the back where the trash went: We would take our break and smoke a fat blunt, timed to my boss being gone, because he had a set schedule.

I tried selling it too, but I'm never good at selling things. I'm too generous—I'll just end up giving it to you. If you even try to bargain with me, I am, yeah, you know what, just take it. I don't have patience. Or I'd smoke it. Though one time my friend gave me some bad weed to sell, and there were these tobacco-flavoring drops they had at smoke shops on West Fourth Street in Manhattan. We started putting that on bad weed, to make it smell like strawberries. It was terrible, but motherfuckers were loving it. For two or three months we had it bopping, selling that strawberry weed.

I had nerve: I started taking almond extract and honey and diluting it with water in a spray bottle, then I'd put that on the weed and put the weed on the light; I thought that it would crystallize and dry up. I don't know what my thought process was, but I did it. I

thought I was slick, like I was doing some chef shit. And crystals on weed weren't even a thing back then. It did not work. It just stayed soaking wet, but I sold it to this one kid; he wasn't happy, but he bought it, soaking-wet almond-extract tree.

It's hard to even explain the crazy things I used to do for weed: the missions that we would go on, the hours spent playing the waiting game, the trickery.

All this is why my favorite weed is still illegal weed. I like to get it illegally: I mean, I don't think it should be banned or illegal in the first place, but I like obtaining it in a way that is kind of shady. Growing up, we would always see this lady in my building on the third floor named Phyllis waiting outside for someone, and then this car would roll up, she'd get in, say what's up, and then the car would leave. So years later we find that it's the weed cab. You would call somebody at the taxi service and you'd ask for a certain car number, and they would come and drop off the dime—always some bad weed, but cheap. The weed cab was a phenomenal service, totally predating the weed services we have now where you call a number and they come give you the shit.

Now there are legal stores in some cities. More cities all the time. But you never get the very best stuff at those stores. The best stuff is more expensive: I can't get it for free, even me. If I'm going to smoke, I gotta put the best in my lungs, and the best is never at the store. I have to find my way to it. I still like it that way: that not so many people know what's up, that you have a secret with someone, that it's like a game, this thing of ours—the weed Cosa Nostra.

There are several ways to stash weed comfortably and efficiently on your person, such as when you're driving and the cops come and pull up behind you*. Or you're at the park smoking a blunt, and you have a little weed in your pocket and the cops come by. What do you do? Throw the blunt behind some bushes, then take the weed from your pocket and put it where they're not going to find it: Between your nuts or your ass. Never inside your asshole—it's only weed. It's not crack, it's not a gun. You'll just go to jail for the night; it's not worth penetration.

So, take the bag of weed in your hand, make sure it's crumpled up, and put it into your pants: You boof** it. If you have nuts, shove it under your nuts, right by your asshole and your thigh, where it becomes like an apex intersection and it just some-how holds it there. When you remove your hand, swipe your hand on your nuts, if you have them, and you'll no longer have the weed smell on your hand, you'll have the nut smell. So when the cop goes to smell your hand, it's, oh, what the hell is that. Like a bum. Sometimes it's good to have bum nuts. The second way is to throw it between your butt cheeks, right by your butthole, so your butt cheeks naturally grasp what you have to stash.

The bigger the crevasse you have between your cheeks, the better: If you have a giant butt, you could hide several things there. When the cops tell you to spread your legs, you just hold your butt cheeks tight and spread your legs. I also have thick thighs, where it creates this airtight package. But this even works for those without that, like Al. If you want to go diving, go ahead. It's a song and dance: They know it's there. Think about it, does some guy really want to go into the nuts of some random guy

How to Hide Weed

with his bare hand for weed? They don't know where that nut has been. And you can always tell when weed has been in somebody's ass. The same way you see a crumpled up dollar, and you know it's been in crazy places.

I feel like everyone should take a little time in the mirror and practice the movement. It's like dribbling a basketball; if you do it enough you'll get nice. And it might save you a trip inside. Still, you can't do this for a plane anymore because they have those body sensors. For some reason at the airport, even with the body sensors, they always gotta check my nuts when I board an airplane, because I wear my shorts low. When I go through the x-ray machine I pull them up so it doesn't ring off. They make a mockery of me in front of everybody, when they do that reverse karate chop up to my balls. It's seven in the morning, is this necessary? That's why I won't give away my secrets of the plane.

* Unless you're really moving weight, there's no reason to stash weed in the car. Or you can have a special stash spot put in, where if you turn on the right blinker, turn the AC on, honk the horn twice, and put the car into neutral, some door opens and a console slides out so you can fit in whatever you want, usually guns and drugs.

** Boof: To throw weed in your ass as soon as authorities are noticed. Also known as to keister something, as in, when the cops pulled us over on Pennsylvania Avenue, he keistered the bag of drugs so no one would find it, and he really wanted to smoke weed in central booking if he got arrested, which he probably would be, because he also didn't have a license. Boof is penetration — as in anal captivation.

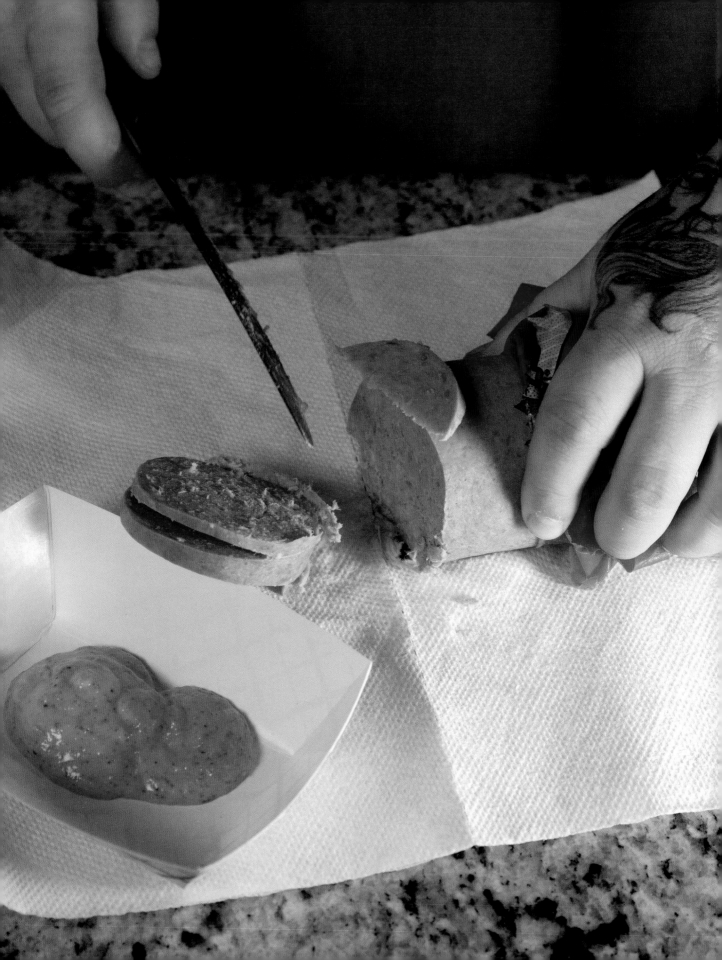

5. The Home Wrecker

Jew salami. Think about it: It's one of the best salamis ever made. Jews know how to make a fucking good salami, if I've ever had one. It's beef, it's Hebrew National, it's, like, fourteen inches long, a massive girth. That's why it's called the home wrecker. It'll wreck any home; it'll send somebody running. There's no recipe. You just peel, slice, eat, at two or three in the morning, perfect timing. A little mustard on the side if you want to get crazy, throw it in a pan if you want to get really nuts. If you want to get reaallllllyyy slick, you know, you can make fire sliders: You could add a little Calabrian chile on it and put it on a Martin's roll. Oof. When I was growing up, they had to stop bringing the salami around my house, because of course I'm going to eat it, I want it. That's another one of those things, like cereal, that has one of those difficult wrappers that people could hear when you're rustling it, so you're letting everyone know what you're doing. There were always twelve people in my house, so of course somebody's going to see me eat the salami. It's not that I am sneaking it; it just makes a lot of noise.

6. Lester

My mom used to really, really, really love weed. She even used to let the kids smoke weed in the house, me and my friends, so we wouldn't get in trouble. As soon as my mother found out I'd started smoking weed, she let me start smoking in the house. I came home stoned out of my mind, and she's like, *Are you fucking stoned out of your mind?* I just told her: *Mom, I am.* She's like, *Cool. You can smoke here if you want.* Then after everyone else went home, when I'd be fiending out for weed, I'd ask my mother for weed, and her connect was our next-door neighbor named Lester.

Lester lived directly across the way from us. All my life Lester was the one always smoking the weed on our floor, fucking stoned out of his mind, gray hair pulled back into a ponytail, hopping into his Honda Accord. He was an accountant, a Jew, an old hippie dealer, not a street dealer. He grew up in the same apartment right there, same as my mother. Neither ever moved. It's a great neighborhood–that's what my mother always says: *It's a great neighborhood.*

I'd say, *Mom, can you get me some treats, can you get me something?* You know I'd bug her: *Please, please can you get me something. Please holler at Lester.* So finally she goes into her room, acts like she's making a phone call to Lester. She goes, *All right, Lester's going to leave it underneath the rug outside the door.* So she would go out there in the hallway and act like he left it there under the rug for her, do this whole spiel, just to make me think it was coming from Lester. Lester was her connection, but she had the weed in her possession the whole time.

She was always hiding things from me: Like I told you in the last book, she'd always hide food. She would hide the cookies from me because I'd be uncontrollable. Trust me, I looked for that weed when she wasn't home: I searched her room, I was sick, I searched everything. She always kept it on her, because she knew it would be glommed, a.k.a. I'd smoke it all.

My mother and Lester also shared space in the garage. I used to always sit in my mother's space smoking weed, and it became a hot spot because I would do it every night: Everyone knew about it, that I was blowing down huge blunts in there. Then motherfuckers started coming through trying to play music, usually on the computer speakers with a little split, plugged into a mini CD Player. The rest of my neighborhood doesn't play that: They're like yentas, all looking out the window. I remember I went out on my own fire escape one time to smoke, and they called the cops on me. It's ridiculous. And it's also why you always need a hub (see page 16).

MOMMA WAS A ROLLING STONE

IT WAS 4/20. MY MOM WAS AT MY HOUSE AND SHE WAS LIKE—

WOO-HOO! I REALLY WANT TO GET HIGH!

I DON'T WANT TO SMOKE THOUGH!

—POKE—

SO I SAID—

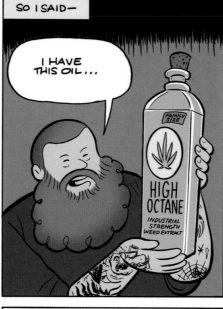

I HAVE THIS OIL...

FAMILY SIZE

HIGH OCTANE

INDUSTRIAL STRENGTH WEED EXTRACT

IT WAS REALLY STRONG OIL. I GOT IT FROM SEATTLE— REFINE SEATTLE, FROM X-TRACTED

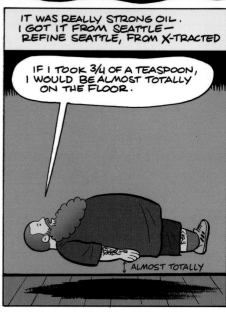

IF I TOOK 3/4 OF A TEASPOON, I WOULD BE ALMOST TOTALLY ON THE FLOOR.

↓ ALMOST TOTALLY

SO I GAVE MY MOTHER JUST A LITTLE NIBBLE OF THE FRONT OF A SPOON.

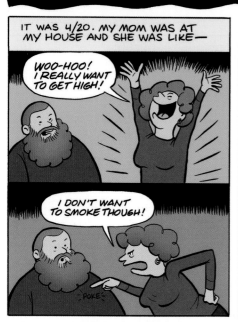

ENLARGED 1000%

WE WERE CHILLING FOR A MINUTE—

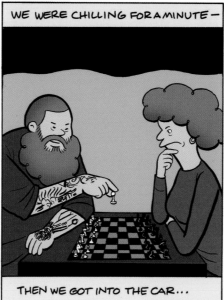

THEN WE GOT INTO THE CAR...

I WAS DRIVING HER HOME, I HAVE THE MUSIC ON OR WHATEVER—

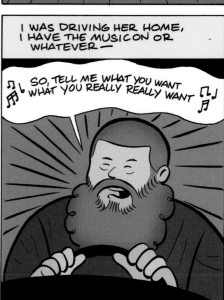

🎵 SO, TELL ME WHAT YOU WANT WHAT YOU REALLY REALLY WANT 🎵

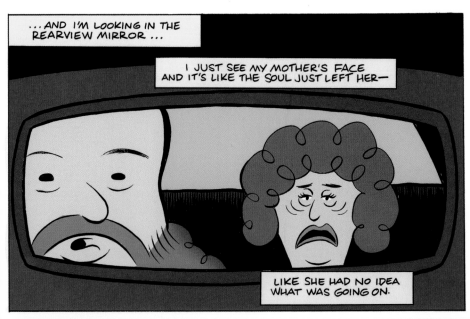

...AND I'M LOOKING IN THE REARVIEW MIRROR...

I JUST SEE MY MOTHER'S FACE AND IT'S LIKE THE SOUL JUST LEFT HER—

LIKE SHE HAD NO IDEA WHAT WAS GOING ON.

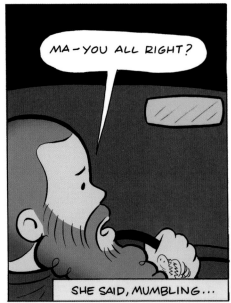

MA—YOU ALL RIGHT?

SHE SAID, MUMBLING...

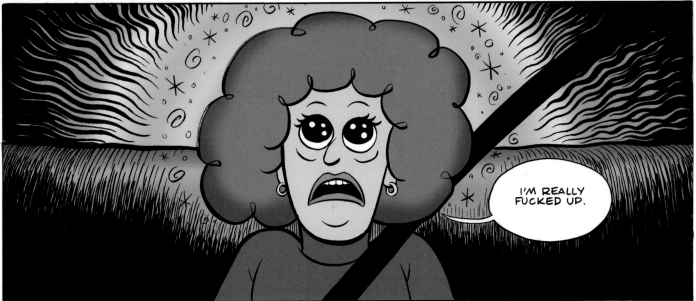

I'M REALLY FUCKED UP.

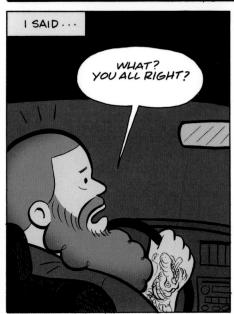

I SAID...

WHAT? YOU ALL RIGHT?

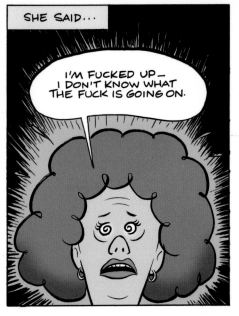

SHE SAID...

I'M FUCKED UP—I DON'T KNOW WHAT THE FUCK IS GOING ON.

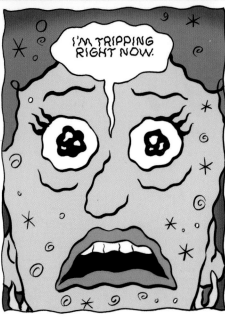

I'M TRIPPING RIGHT NOW.

THE STRONGEST FEELING SHE'S EVER HAD IN HER LIFE. SAYING FUNNY THINGS...

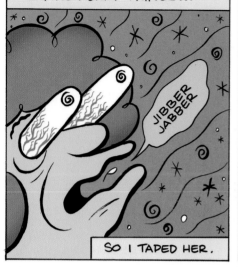

JIBBER JABBER

SO I TAPED HER.

IT'S ON THE ALBUM — I SAID:

TELL THEM HOW HIGH YOU ARE.

SHE SAID:

I DON'T WANT TO TELL ANYONE.

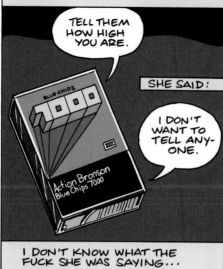

I DON'T KNOW WHAT THE FUCK SHE WAS SAYING...

SO THEN I DROPPED HER OFF. I LITERALLY HAD TO CARRY MY MOTHER UPSTAIRS.

WHERE AM I?

HUFF PUFF

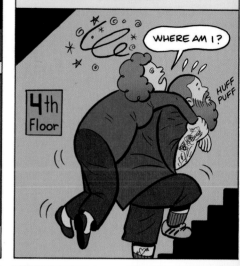

SHE COULDN'T WALK — I HAD TO FUCKING CARRY HER UPSTAIRS AND PUT HER TO BED.

THERE YOU GO— NOW LET'S TAKE OFF YOUR SHOES.

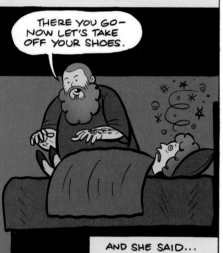

AND SHE SAID...

DON'T TAKE MY SHOES OFF!

DON'T FUCKING TAKE MY SHOES OFF!

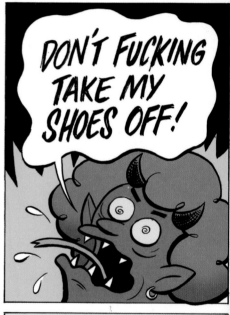

...BECAUSE SHE WAS SCARED IF SHE GOT UP, SHE'D FALL IF SHE DIDN'T HAVE HER SHOES ON.

AAAUGHH!

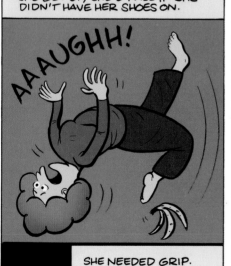

SHE NEEDED GRIP.

SO — SHE SLEPT FOR A DAY AND A HALF IN HER SHOES. SHE SAYS SHE WASN'T FULLY TOGETHER FOR 3 DAYS. THEN SHE WAS LIKE:

WOW— THAT WAS A TRIP!

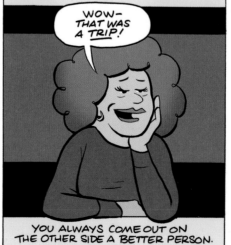

YOU ALWAYS COME OUT ON THE OTHER SIDE A BETTER PERSON.

YOU MADE IT THROUGH. YOU KNOW YOU'RE A FUCKING WARRIOR—

THE BODY CAN TAKE A LICKING AND KEEP ON TICKING—

I'LL TELL YOU THAT.

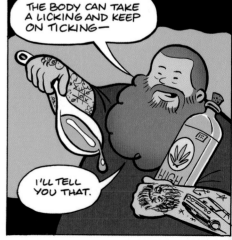

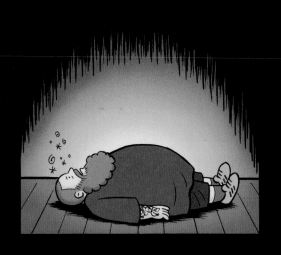

7. My Mom's Cheesecake with Extra Crust and Homemade Jam

This is The Cheesecake. Mama's cheesecake. I've seen my mother make these cheesecakes for people for my entire life. People would just order them from her, and she would charge them $30. Which is, I think, not enough: She pretty much paid $30 for all the ingredients to make a cheesecake. I felt like she could have had one of these businesses just selling cheesecakes. They're that good. I really haven't tasted one better than this recipe, a result of years of tinkering by my mother. I bring a slightly more proper way to mix things and this and that and use fresh lime juice whereas she uses Rose's. She also always does the crust just on the bottom, never around, but I like a crust all the way around so it kind of encases the cheesecake. The crust tastes amazing, plus, it looks cool. You could also add a little whipped cream on top, and you could add any preserves you had. Cheesecakes are one of the greatest things in life, and making one is like riding a bike for me. I'll never forget how.

Makes 1 9-inch (23-cm) cheesecake

1 stick (4 ounce/113 g) unsalted butter, softened, plus extra for greasing the pan
2 sleeves graham crackers
2 ¼ cups (250 g) granulated sugar, divided
3 8-ounce (226-g) packages Philadelphia cream cheese, at room temperature
½ cup (115 g) sour cream
1 tablespoon freshly squeezed lime juice
1 tablespoon vanilla extract
4 large eggs

FOR SERVING, OPTIONAL
Homemade jam (page 32)
Whipped cream (page 35, step 2)
Really good extra virgin olive oil (page 183)

1. Preheat the oven to 350°F (175°C), and grease a 9-inch (23-cm) springform pan with butter and set it aside.

2. In a mixing bowl, crush the graham crackers with the softened stick of butter and ¼ cup (52 g) of the sugar until it is well blended. Pat this mixture into the springform pan, using the back of a large spoon or a glass, so that it flattens out and goes all the way up the sides of the pan. It's OK if the edges are uneven and rough.

3. Bake the crust for 10 minutes, then set it aside to cool completely.

4. Put the remaining 2 cups (430 g) sugar and cream cheese in the bowl of a stand mixer fitted with the paddle attachment and beat on medium-low speed until very creamy and soft. Slowly add the sour cream, the lime juice, and the vanilla, beating until all are well mixed.

5. Add the eggs one at a time, beating after each addition until well blended, making sure to scrape down the sides of the bowl.

6. Use a spatula to transfer the mixture to the cooled crust.

7. Bake the cheesecake for 40 minutes, then turn the oven off and open the door slightly.

8. Leave the cheesecake in the oven with the door open for 30 minutes, then remove it to a rack to cool completely to room temperature.

9. Refrigerate the cheesecake until fully chilled—several hours or even overnight—before you slice it.

10. Serve each slice topped with homemade jam, whipped cream, and olive oil.

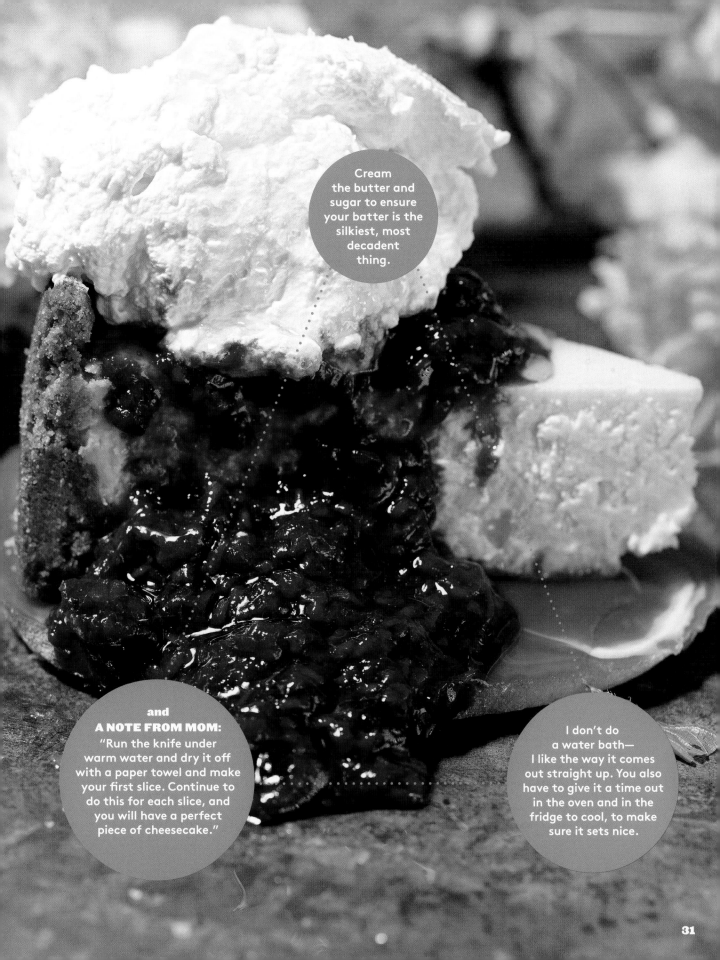

Cream the butter and sugar to ensure your batter is the silkiest, most decadent thing.

and
A NOTE FROM MOM:
"Run the knife under warm water and dry it off with a paper towel and make your first slice. Continue to do this for each slice, and you will have a perfect piece of cheesecake."

I don't do a water bath—I like the way it comes out straight up. You also have to give it a time out in the oven and in the fridge to cool, to make sure it sets nice.

HOMEMADE JAMS

I like to make homemade jams from whatever bags of good organic frozen fruit I have in my freezer and serve them with all kinds of things: cheesecake, fried cheese, bread and butter, or milk bun sandwiches.

Peach Jam

Makes about 2 cups

2 tablespoons olive oil
4 whole dried red Calabrian chiles
1 10-ounce (285-g) bag frozen sliced organic peaches
1 tablespoon granulated sugar

1. Heat the olive oil in a medium saucepan over medium-high heat. Add the chiles and let them cook until they are puffed, fragrant, and charred.

2. Add the frozen peaches, the sugar, and ½ cup (120 ml) of water and let it come to a simmer.

3. Let the mixture cook over medium heat, stirring occasionally, until it breaks down and becomes jam-like, about 15 to 20 minutes. This will keep in the fridge for about a week.

Strawberry Jam

Makes about 2 cups

1 10-ounce (285-g) bag frozen strawberries
1 tablespoon granulated sugar
1 small handful fresh mint leaves, washed and dried

1. Add the frozen strawberries, the sugar, and ½ cup (120 ml) of water to a medium saucepan over medium-high heat and let everything come to a simmer.

2. Add the mint leaves and let the mixture cook, stirring occasionally, until it breaks down and becomes jam-like, about 15 to 20 minutes. This will keep in the fridge for about a week.

Mango Jam

Makes about 2 cups

1 10-ounce (285-g) bag frozen mango
1 tablespoon granulated sugar
1 tablespoon Indian amchoor (dried mango powder)

1. Add the frozen mango, the sugar, and ½ cup (120 ml) of water to a medium saucepan over medium-high heat and let everything come to a simmer.

2. Let the mixture cook, stirring occasionally, until it breaks down and becomes jam-like, about 15 to 20 minutes, then stir in the mango powder. This will keep in the fridge for about a week.

Berry Jam

Makes about 4 cups

1 10-ounce (285-g) bag frozen blueberries
1 10-ounce (285-g) bag frozen raspberries
2 tablespoons granulated sugar

1. Add the frozen fruit, the sugar, and 1 cup (240 ml) of water to a medium saucepan over medium-high heat and let everything come to a simmer.

2. Let the mixture cook, stirring occasionally, until it breaks down and becomes jam-like, about 30 minutes. This will keep in the fridge for about a week.

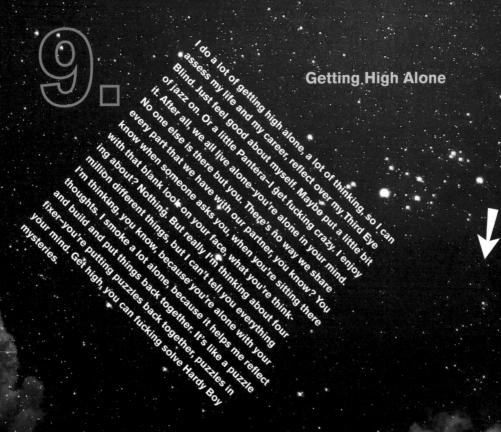

The Celestial Origins of Weed

8.

Supposedly cannabis was an ancient gift to the first humans from the goddess of the dog stars: Sirius, the brightest star in the night sky and part of a constellation known as the Greater Dog, and Procyon, part of a constellation called the Lesser Dog. In Greek, cannabis means "two dogs." This is one reason why my show where I smoked weed and watched *Ancient Aliens* was called *Traveling the Stars: I believe we were all put here at the same time, that weed actually helped man and woman evolve,*

9.

Getting High Alone

I do a lot of getting high alone, a lot of thinking, so I can assess my life and my career, reflect over my Third Eye Blind. Just feel good about myself. Maybe put a little bit of jazz on. Or a little Pantera—I get fucking crazy. I enjoy it. After all, we all live alone—you're alone in your mind. No one else is there but you. There's no way we share every part that we have with our partner, you know? You know when someone asks you, when you're sitting there with that blank look on your face, what you're think- ing about? Nothing. But really I'm thinking about four million different things, but I can't tell you everything I'm thinking, you know, because you're alone with your thoughts. I smoke a lot alone, because it helps me reflect and build and put things back together. It's like a puzzle fixer—you're putting puzzles back together, puzzles in your mind. Get high, you can fucking solve Hardy Boy mysteries.

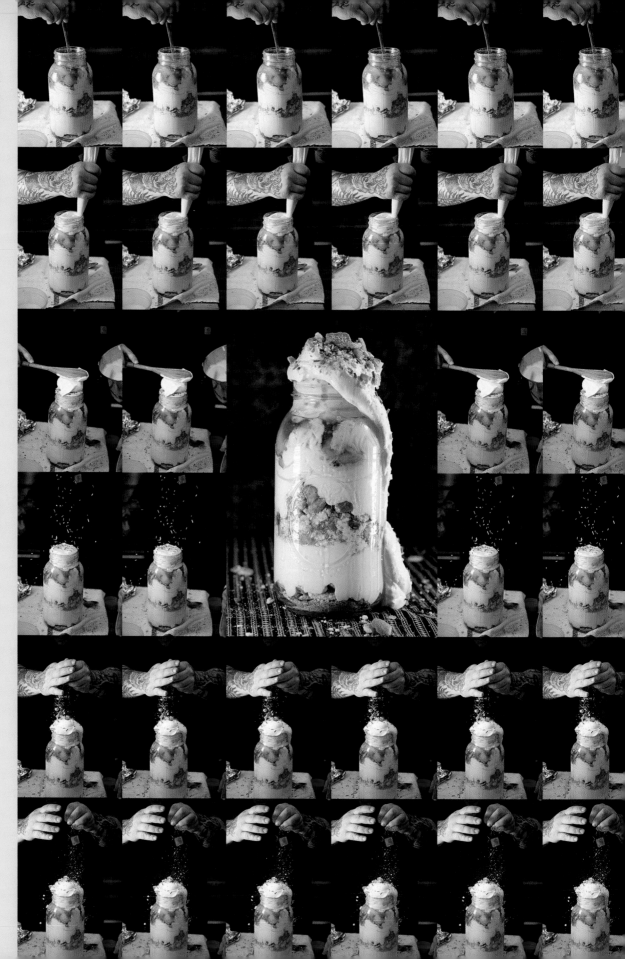

10. Banana Pudding

Are you fucking crazy? Of course we're going to have the banana pudding. We're just going to doctor up the stuff from the box with crazy amounts of gently whipped cream and caramelized bananas and Nilla wafers crushed with melted butter. Yes, you could make the pudding from scratch, but this is just as good. No, this is better: It takes seconds to set up, then you go in, and it tastes like you made real pudding. Pro tip: Top this with really good, grassy-green olive oil (like California Olive Ranch) and a light hand with the sprinkles. The olive oil really picks up notes of green banana—it's amazing. And the sprinkles? Next. Who makes banana pudding with sprinkles?

Serves 6–8

3 small (3.4 ounce/96 g) boxes Jell-O banana cream instant pudding and pie filling

4 cups (1 quart/L) whole milk

4 cups (1 quart/L) heavy cream

1¼ tablespoons granulated sugar

16 ounces (2 sticks/226 g) unsalted butter

1 box (11 ounces/311 g) Nilla wafers

4 ripe bananas

¼ cup (67 g) brown sugar

Pinch ground cinnamon

Extra virgin olive oil, optional garnish

Multicolor sprinkles, optional garnish

1. In a large mixing bowl whisk the dry pudding with the milk. Set the bowl in the refrigerator to cool.

2. To make whipped cream, in another large mixing bowl whip the heavy cream with the sugar with a whisk or hand mixer just until soft peaks form.

3. Gently fold 3 cups (720 ml) of the whipped cream into the pudding mixture so that it is well incorporated. Fold in more as needed until the pudding is light and fluffy (and tastes like homemade pudding, not like something out of a box). Put the pudding and any leftover whipped cream in the refrigerator.

4. In a large skillet, melt one of the sticks of butter and pour it into the bottom of a baking dish or another mixing bowl. Use your hands to crumble about ⅔ of the box of Nilla wafers into the baking dish. Stir the cookies into the butter with a spoon or spatula until it forms a loose crumble. Set this aside.

5. Heat the second stick of butter in the same skillet over medium heat. Peel the bananas, cut them in half (not lengthwise), and add them to the skillet when the butter begins to bubble. Sprinkle the brown sugar and the cinnamon over the top.

6. Cook the bananas, swirling them in the pan or moving them around with a spoon, until both are coated in the butter–brown sugar mixture. Let it cook until the mixture begins to look like lava and starts to crinkle up, then remove the pan from the heat.

7. To serve the banana pudding, you can make one large dessert or several small ones: Put down a few inches of Nilla wafer–crumble, then top it with a few more of caramelized bananas, making sure to get some sauce. Add a few hefty spoonfuls of chilled banana pudding, then top with a little more crumble. (If you are using a tall container, repeat these layers one or two more times as needed.)

8. Then top the whole thing with a generous dollop of whipped cream—pressing down the layers if need be to make the whipped cream fit—and finish with a drizzle of olive oil, sprinkles, and a few crumbled plain Nilla wafers.

11.

Fast Food

Fast food goes hand in hand with driving around and smoking blunts (see Cruising Around While Getting High, page 114). You don't ever have to get out of the car: You just ride around, smoke, eat your food, and throw the wrappers in a garbage can from the car. When you're out late at night, going around fucking high as fuck, you're so tempted by those bright lights on the boulevard: the arches, the big shining light with the little girl with the pigtails on the sign, the castle in white.

The Subway card was big deal, back in the day. It was the first of its kind. We used to be stoned, play handball, then go get Subway on Queens Boulevard over by the courthouse. With the card, after buying a certain number of sandwiches, you'd eventually get a free sub. And dudes coveted that card: You carried it around like it was your ID.* We used to get the veggie combo, 'cause it was cheap, and we would go to the store and steal the cold cuts to put on it. You'd go steal the cold cuts first. A pound on the sandwich. Just like they do at Subway, lay it in in that pre-sliced layer. The thing is, in certain supermarkets the deli's in the back, and for some reason they trust you enough to walk to the front to pay. At least back then they did—no cameras at the time. Two seconds into the aisle that shit's already gone, already in my underwear by then. Or you would get a whole sandwich and throw it down your leg. We would have a pound of honey turkey on the sandwich, roast beef, ham, whatever. When the Boar's Head jerk chicken came out, that was what was fucking popping off. The veggie combo was three dollars, and it came with a soda. At the Subway on Queens Boulevard you could go up and get as much soda as you wanted. Remember those? But that was early days, before all the fuckery with Jared.

I fuck with everything from Popeye's. I really like the tenders. I love the spicy breast. I love a breast and a wing. That's my combo. We were talking about the piece of breast— the extra little niblet—on the wing; there's another piece of breast on the wing, so you could get two of those, and that shit's satisfying. It's tremendous with the honey biscuit. Of course, you get the biscuit and

the mashed potatoes. The dirty mashed potatoes; they put the same dirty in the mashed potatoes that they do in the rice. So it's like a sausage-gravy-giblets-gibberish type thing. Popeye's chicken is better than KFC's chicken, for sure. The original recipe for KFC is always soggy, but it still has that flavor, and I like that flavor. Plus, the way it gets soggy is both disgusting and great. If you order the spicy, it's crunchier.

I love Sbarro. That's the pizza I grew up on going to the mall; it's straight mall pizza. That was the first time I saw the double slice, with the bottom and the top crust, both with toppings. That was the most poppin' shit in Queens Center Mall. I fuck with the mall: When I was younger, one of my favorite pastimes was walking around the Roosevelt Field mall. Just the circle of food concessions, just get a sample from each person. You'd be in your car, you'd be stoned—*let's get out here.* Because you always needed somewhere to go. *What are we going to do today? Let's fucking drive to the mall while we're smoking. And we need to smoke on the way back, too.*

McDonald's? I'm not going to lie, not too long ago I went through the drive-through and got a sundae real quick. I was on my way to my studio, and I was stressed out, it was, like, three in the morning. I was like, fuck it, made the mad sharp turn through the drive-through, hit the gas, *errrrkkk,* that sound your tires make when you stop really sharp at the speaker. Usually they don't have ice cream machines running at night, but I took a shot. It was summertime. So I got me a fucking fudge sundae. I've never had a shake, only a McFlurry or a sundae. The McFlurry you gotta get with extra M&M's, so you're essentially just eating ice-cream-coated M&M's. And once in a while I would run and get a mozzarella stick from Burger King, but ever since they tried to change their fry to have some crunch to it, it pissed me off—really upsetting.

We also recently ordered a fucking hundred dollars' worth of Taco Bell after a show in Connecticut. It was two in the morning, we were starving, and it was the only thing open somewhere off the highway, so we

pulled up and ordered everything. They were pissed. And it took an hour—we were waiting outside the Taco Bell for an hour, watching old UFC fights in the car, specifically the one where Francis Ngannou fights Alistair Overeem on December 2, 2017. Ngannou just fucking knocked Overeem to the fucking moon, and Overeem is one of the greatest mixed martial arts fighters of all time, a heavyweight champion from the Netherlands. Francis Ngannou is a new dude from Cameroon fighting out of Paris, and that knockout was unbelievable. But then when the food finally came out, it was cold as fuck, soggy, and wet. (We ate it all.)

P.S. It can damage the urethra. (Also if you run the water while you're pissing, it makes you piss harder.)

* I still have a Key Food card from my old neighborhood attached to my key chain. You know, you bring the card to get the savings. They scan it, $3 would come off, and you're like, *ohhkay.*

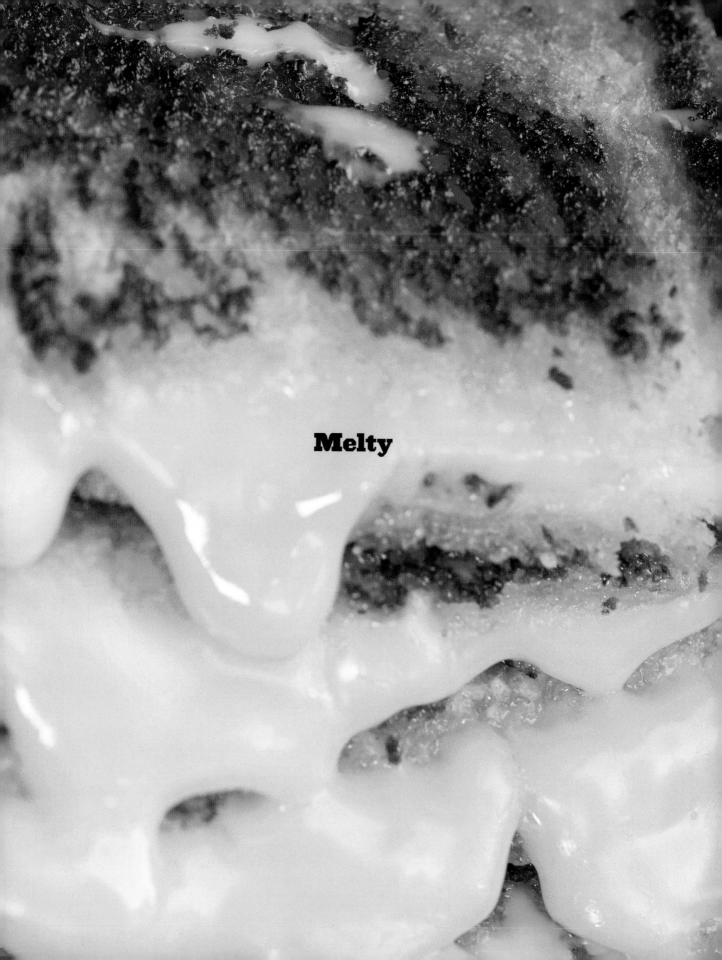
Melty

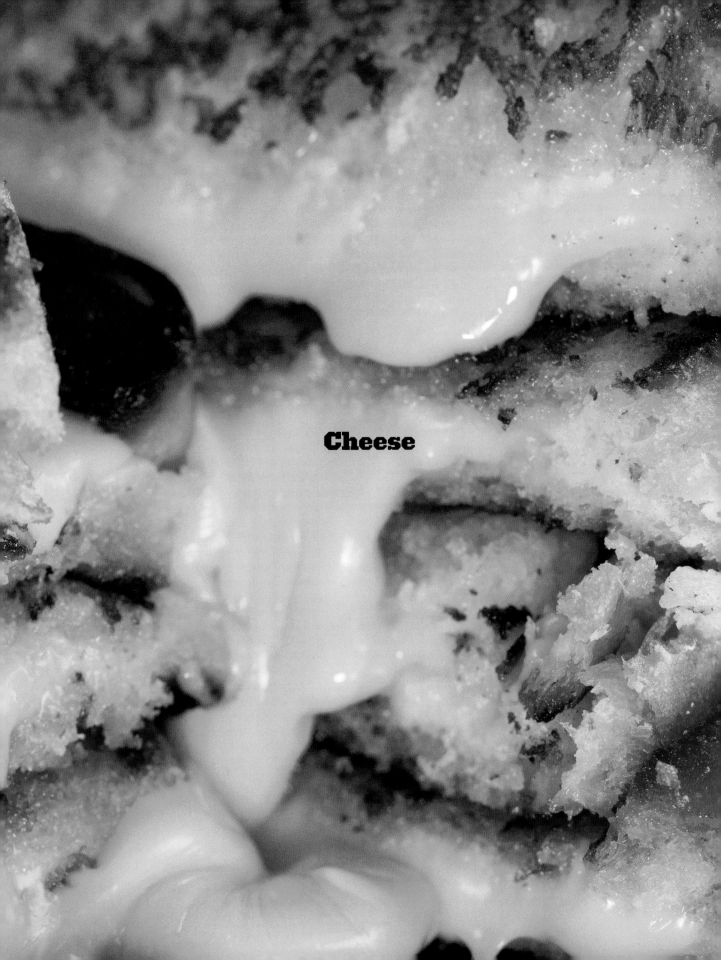

Cheese

12.
Grilled Cheese

Who hasn't had a grilled cheese sandwich before in their life? Grilled cheese is as American as baseball. Grilled cheese is also spiritual. I usually just go straight-up American cheese, specifically Land O'Lakes, as there is nothing that melts better than Land O'Lakes. It's a beautifully made American cheese. It's not always American cheese on my grilled cheese, but my natural instinct is usually to go white bread, American cheese, and ketchup on the side, 100 percent. I'm a purist.

Makes 1 sandwich, can be multiplied as needed

2 slices white Wonder Bread
2 slices Land O'Lakes or Boar's Head American cheese
2 tablespoons extra virgin olive oil
2 tablespoons unsalted butter at room temperature
Ketchup to taste

1. Put the American cheese between the two slices of bread.

2. Heat the olive oil in a skillet over medium-high heat.

3. Butter one side of the sandwich. Place the buttered side down in the olive oil. While the bottom side cooks, spread the other side of the sandwich with butter.

4. Flip the sandwich when the bottom is dark golden brown and crunchy, which should take a few minutes, then let the other side cook until the bottom is dark golden brown and crunchy.

5. Cut in half and eat immediately with ketchup on the side.

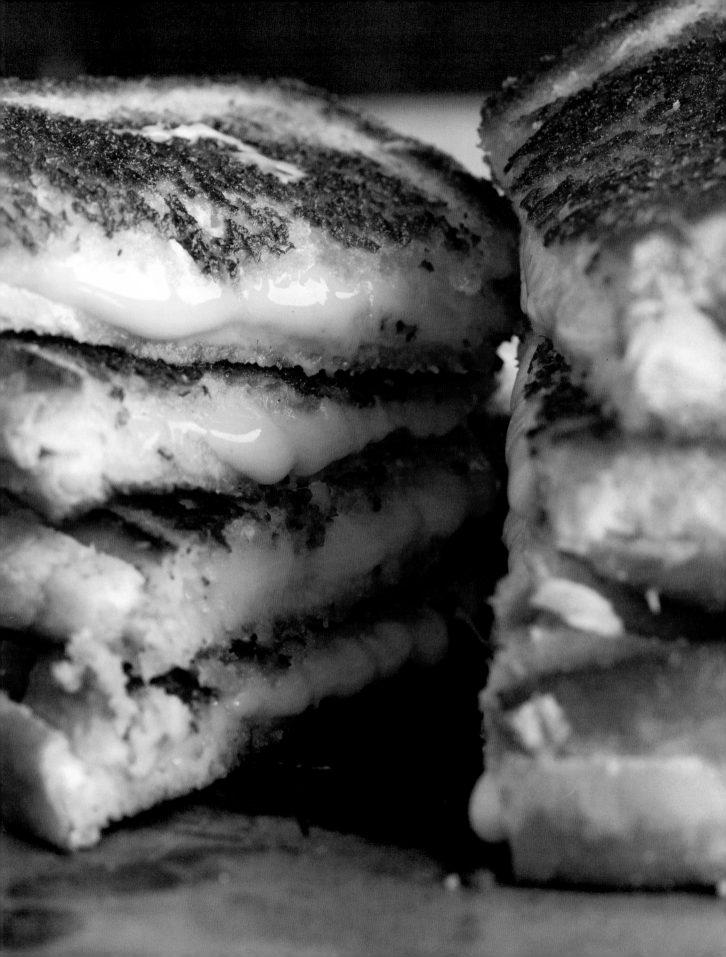

13. Egg and Cheese on a Roll

I usually don't like eggs cooked by other people. I have to make the egg; I just don't trust anyone with the egg. For a fried-egg sandwich, I like almost deep-frying the egg, to the point when it gets really fucking crunchy on the outside. And I prefer it on a good challah roll, preferably homemade. I'm going to be honest with you: I hate most breakfast—Benedicts and shit like that—but I do like an egg and cheese.

HOW TO MAKE A PERFECT HOMEMADE EGG AND CHEESE ON A ROLL:

1. Make the challah from my previous book, *F*ck, That's Delicious*. But instead of dividing the dough into three ropes to make a braid, divide it into twelve even pieces. Let them rise another 10 minutes, then brush them with softened butter and sprinkle them with sesame seeds. Bake until golden-brown at the same temperature as the original recipe, about 25 to 30 minutes. Brush them with butter again and let them cool on a rack.

2. When the challah rolls are ready, split open a roll and layer a few slices of good American cheese on the top bun. Set this aside.

3. Fry an egg in plenty of olive oil over medium-high heat, almost like you are shallow-frying it. If you're not sure how much olive oil to use, err on the side of a lot. Let the egg cook until the edges are lacy and golden-brown.

4. Put the egg on the roll, slather the egg with sea salt, freshly ground pepper, and Heinz ketchup to your liking, and close it up.

LET ME GET AN EGG AND CHEESE ON A ROLL, SALT, PEPPER, KETCHUP.

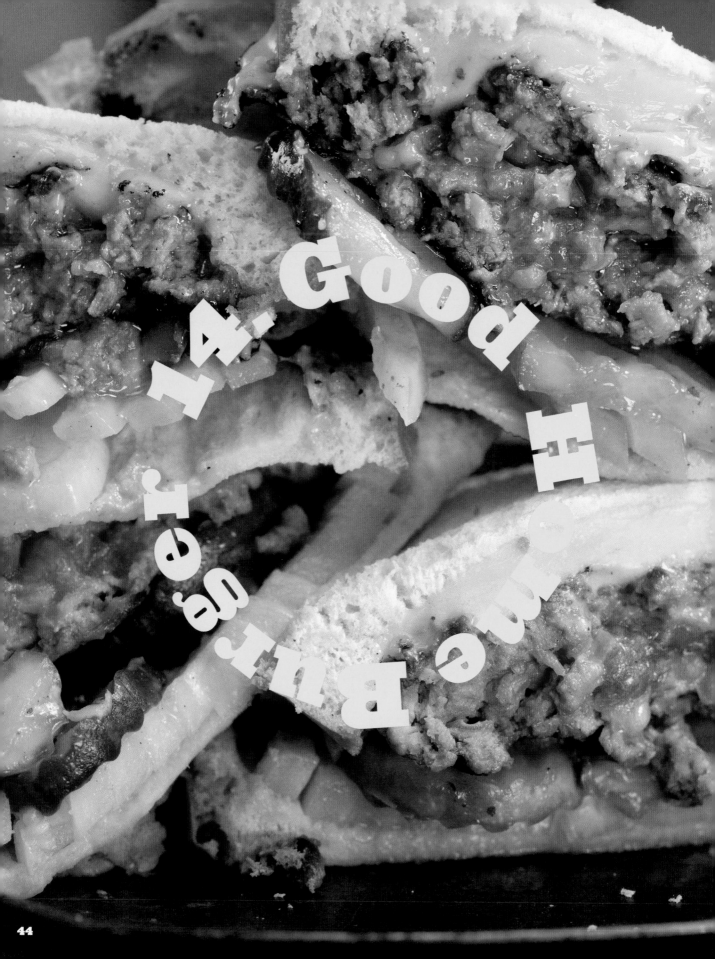

14. Good Home Burger

This is a good home burger on white bread, like my Albanian grandmother, my nonna, used to make me, though she would usually add parsley and onion. It wasn't till I was much older that I found out that hamburgers do not have parsley and onion in them and that what she was making was Balkan *pljeskavica*. This is a simple burger, but details count: To make a good home burger, the meat should be at least 70 percent fat to lean, the bread should preferably be Wonder Bread, the cheese should preferably be Land O'Lakes or Boar's Head, and the bread-and-butter pickles should not be Vlasic. I genuinely don't fuck with Vlasic. (My mother generally had many kinds of good pickles in the fridge, because a good Jew always has good pickles in the fridge—sweet dills, half sours, and so on.) You must let the ground beef come to real room temperature. If it hits that hot oil and it's cold, that nice Maillard browning reaction doesn't work. Any cook anywhere knows this, even if they don't really practice it.

Makes 4 burgers

1 pound (454 g) ground beef, at room temperature
2 tablespoons olive oil
Kosher salt to taste
1 white onion, sliced into 1/4-inch (6 mm)-thick rounds
8 slices soft white bread
Bread and butter pickles to taste
8 slices American cheese

1. Form the meat into 4 thin patties, around 1-inch (2.5-cm) thick, and set them aside. Try not to over-work the beef: The patties can be loose, even crumbly. (This is the beauty of the tube. You know those tubes of ground beef you buy from the grocery store? You can just slice one into four perfect burger patties.)

2. Heat the oil in a large skillet until it is screaming hot.

3. Sprinkle the patties on one side with the salt, then place them salt-side down in the pan, pressing them down gently to make sure they are flat on the pan. Sprinkle the other side with salt. (If only two patties fit in the pan, cook two at a time.)

4. Cook each burger for several minutes until it is crusty and deep-brown on one side, then flip it over and cook the other side until it is crusty brown.

5. While the burgers cook, lay one slice of white onion on each of four slices of bread and top the slice of onion with a few pickles.

6. Add two slices of cheese to each patty, and once the cheese has melted, quickly transfer the burger on top of the pickles so that the cheese side still faces up. Add the other slice of bread, then press the whole thing down so you can see a handprint in the bread. (There has to be a handprint.) Serve immediately.

15. Papi Dog

This is one of those magical one-off creations that came to be one day while I was Stoned Beyond Belief. Leftover hot dogs from the Salchipapas on page 106 mixed with leftover Good Home Burger supplies (page 44) plus my new invention of wrapping things in frico-ed American cheese (see page 48 for frico-ing). Did it really happen? We don't know. We do know that for this to be magical, you have to score the hot dog two ways on the diagonal, then fry it so it twists open in a beautiful way. The fried cheese really adds that last little caramelized something.

Makes 1 papi dog, can be multiplied as needed

1 hot dog good enough for Salchipapas (see page 106)
1 teaspoon olive oil
2 slices American cheese
1 slice soft white bread
2 tablespoons diced white onion
2 tablespoons diced bread-and-butter pickles

1. Use a sharp knife to make a series of shallow diagonal scores along the hot dog every inch (2.5 cm) or so down one side, then turn the dog 180 degrees and do the same to the other side.

2. Heat the olive oil in a skillet (you can skip the oil if you use a nonstick pan) to medium high and then add the scored hot dog. Let the dog lightly fry in the oil and fat it releases for a minute or two, turning it often with a fork, until it is golden-brown around the edges and the scores slightly fan out. Remove the hot dog to a plate or a cutting board.

3. Turn the heat to low and lay the two slices of cheese in the skillet so they slightly overlap. Let them cook for a few minutes until they fully melt and begin to brown around the edges. Lay the hot dog down the center of the cheese lengthwise. Use the tines of a fork to gently lift the edges of the fried cheese up and over the dog, almost like you're making a pig in a blanket with cheese.

4. Use a spatula to gently remove the cheese-wrapped dog from the skillet and place it diagonally into the slice of bread.

5. Top with onion and pickle and go in.

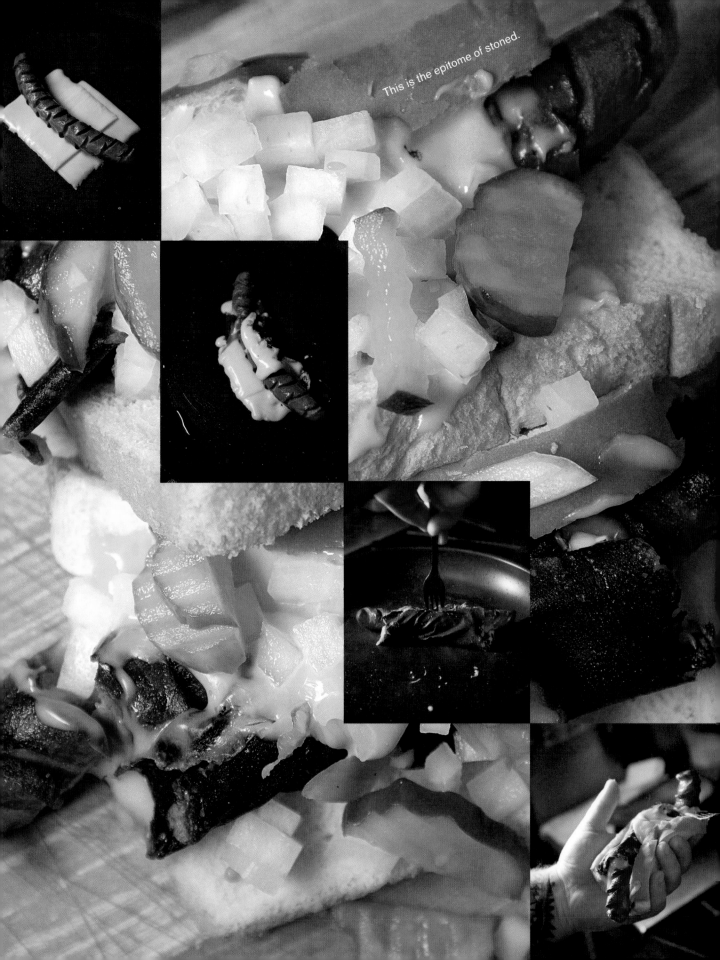

This is the epitome of stoned.

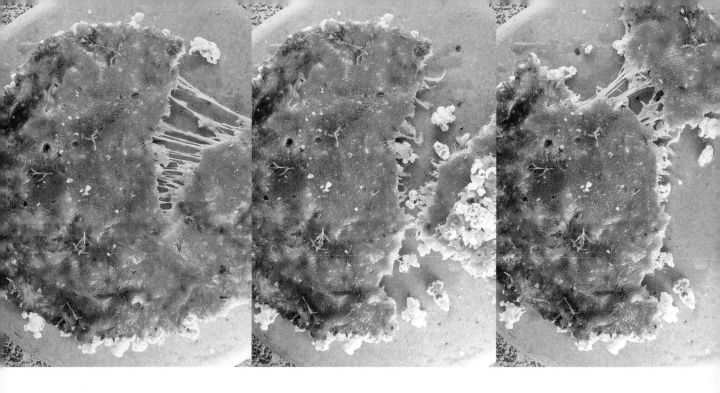

16. Frico Popcorn

Jacques Pepin is the man, one of my all-time favorite chefs. He's been teaching me how to cook forever, and he taught me how to make this when he came on my show *Untitled*, though he used fancier cheese. Frico is Northern Italian—it's cheese shredded and cooked in a thin layer until it is all crunch and caramelization, like a giant round wafer of crunchy cheese. Then you just lay in the popcorn and flip it over on a plate. I make the frico layer extra thick. The red bag of plain salted popcorn from Popcorn, Indiana—that's the good kind to buy.

Serves 4

2 tablespoons olive oil
2 garlic cloves, minced
1 teaspoon Aleppo chili powder or crumbled Calabrian chile flakes
1 teaspoon freshly ground black pepper
¼ teaspoon dried thyme
¼ cup (31 g) shredded sharp Cheddar cheese
¼ cup (31 g) shredded whole-milk mozzarella
2 cups popped popcorn

1. Heat the olive oil in a skillet over medium heat and add the garlic. Let it cook, stirring often, for a few minutes until it is soft and translucent. Add the chiles, black pepper, and thyme.

2. Sprinkle the cheeses evenly over the skillet. Let them melt for several minutes without touching or stirring them—when they begin to fry and crisp around the edges, lay the popcorn down in a single layer into the skillet, gently pressing to embed it into the cheese.

3. Turn off the heat. Once the cheese has cooled completely, invert the frico popcorn onto a plate. Rip off pieces as desired and enjoy.

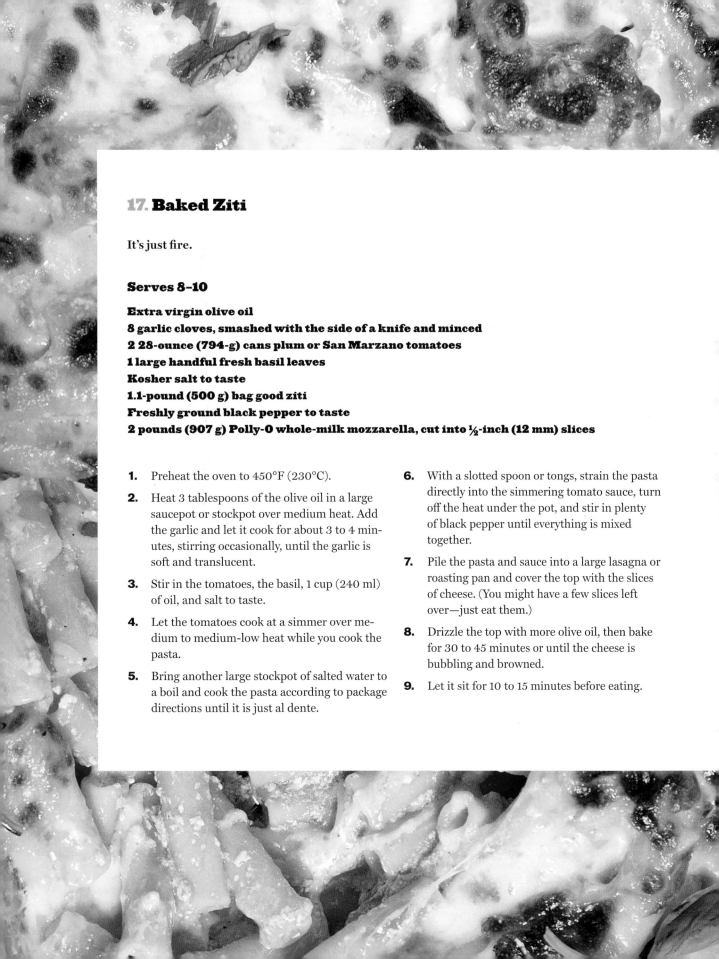

17. Baked Ziti

It's just fire.

Serves 8–10

Extra virgin olive oil
8 garlic cloves, smashed with the side of a knife and minced
2 28-ounce (794-g) cans plum or San Marzano tomatoes
1 large handful fresh basil leaves
Kosher salt to taste
1.1-pound (500 g) bag good ziti
Freshly ground black pepper to taste
2 pounds (907 g) Polly-O whole-milk mozzarella, cut into ½-inch (12 mm) slices

1. Preheat the oven to 450°F (230°C).

2. Heat 3 tablespoons of the olive oil in a large saucepot or stockpot over medium heat. Add the garlic and let it cook for about 3 to 4 minutes, stirring occasionally, until the garlic is soft and translucent.

3. Stir in the tomatoes, the basil, 1 cup (240 ml) of oil, and salt to taste.

4. Let the tomatoes cook at a simmer over medium to medium-low heat while you cook the pasta.

5. Bring another large stockpot of salted water to a boil and cook the pasta according to package directions until it is just al dente.

6. With a slotted spoon or tongs, strain the pasta directly into the simmering tomato sauce, turn off the heat under the pot, and stir in plenty of black pepper until everything is mixed together.

7. Pile the pasta and sauce into a large lasagna or roasting pan and cover the top with the slices of cheese. (You might have a few slices left over—just eat them.)

8. Drizzle the top with more olive oil, then bake for 30 to 45 minutes or until the cheese is bubbling and browned.

9. Let it sit for 10 to 15 minutes before eating.

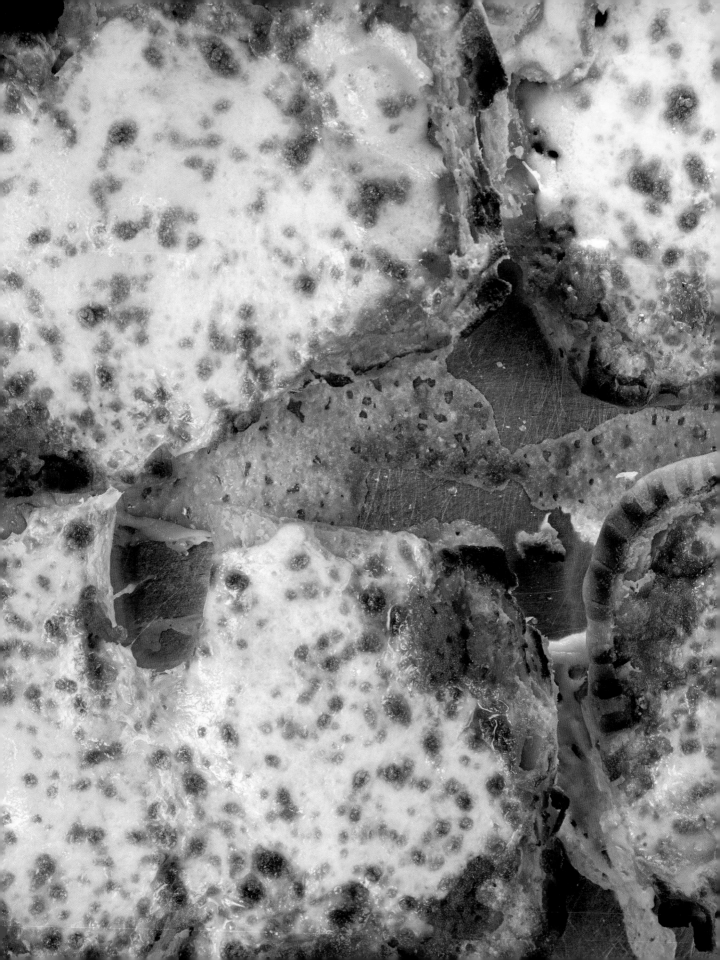

18. Jamaican Beef Patty with Cheese

The New York City pizzeria is where you get the Jamaican patty with mozzarella, and sometimes pepperoni too. They cut it open, they put it in tinfoil, and they put the mozzarella on there, and then they heat it again in the pizza oven. The motherfucker who thought of that was 100 percent stoned out of their fucking mind. Who else would think to do that other than somebody working at a pizzeria, stoned out of their mind? A lot of the greatest creations were made when someone was stoned.

HOW TO MAKE A PATTY WITH CHEESE:

1. Bake frozen Jamaican beef patties as per package directions.

2. Split the patty open lengthwise, like a clam, so there's a little bit of meat on both sides.

3. Sprinkle the tops generously with grated mozzarella.

4. Broil them until the cheese is browned and bubbly, about 5 minutes.

5. Serve open-faced, with hot sauce and a Coke.

19. Biscuits with Cheese and Guava Paste

You see what we're doing here? We're taking something crappy from the store and we're making it amazing.* You load up those pop-a-can biscuits with butter and mild cheese and guava, and they come out just like the *pastelitos de guayaba y queso*—the puff pastry with guava and cheese—from all over Latin America. Popping the pressurized cardboard can is actually the hardest part—it's terrifying, it never works. This is the best they can do now? This is the best in biscuit can technology?
*See also Fried Pizza, page 104.

HOW TO MAKE *PASTELITOS DE GUAYABA Y QUESO* WITH PILLSBURY GRANDS:

1. Split each biscuit almost all the way open, making a little pouch.

2. Fill the pouch with a thick slice of queso fresco or mozzarella—go crazy, do two slices—and a thick slice of guava paste.

3. Close the biscuit back up, pinching the edges closed. Stretch the dough a little around the bulge, if necessary, if you went with two slices of cheese. It'll look a little messy but will still come out OK.

4. Then top the tops with a thick pat of butter. This is key—and sprinkle them with sesame seeds, if you want to get crazy.

5. Bake them at the temperature specified on the can until the tops are fully browned, at least 10 minutes longer than it says to on the can.

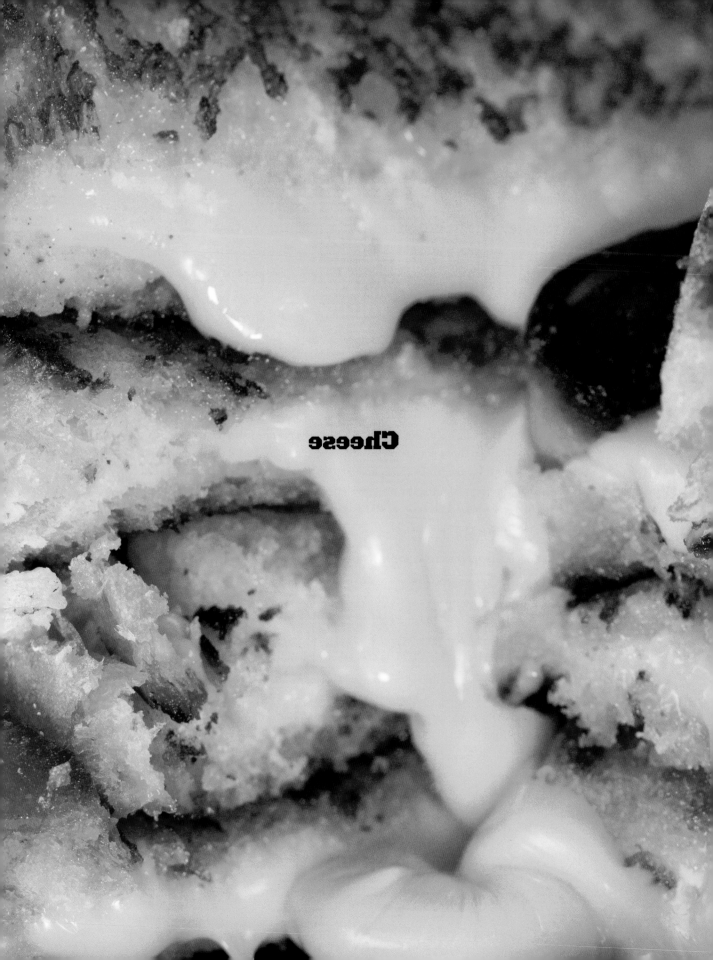

Cheese

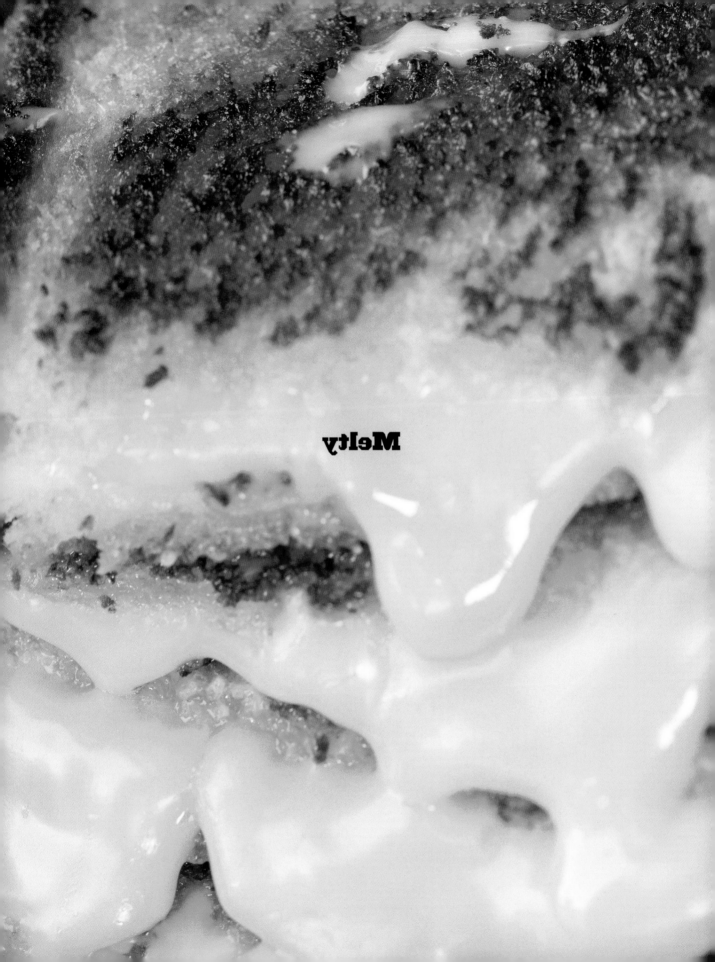

20.

The
Beach

and other Special Places
to Smoke Weed

The beach is always a beautiful place to be: You want to be there at five in the morning or just when the sun is going down. It's usually very, very windy, so it's not the greatest place to smoke, but if you smoke in a little nook somewhere, and then you just hang there, it's fire. I've been on so many beaches around this fucking Earth, just find a nook, or hold the joint in your hand and protect the fire. It's also amazing how much ingenuity we can come up with in order to smoke, how much drive, that we will find a way.

Overlooking water from an elevated aspect.
Anything elevated, looking down on something, that's fire.

Cenotes. Yes, it's a freshwater underground pool, but it is also a cathedral underneath the ground, a cathedral-cave with a humongous, gorgeous underground pool. Cenotes are breathtaking, all the formations down there, and the water is filled with minerals. The water is clear, it's freezing cold, it's pure, and some weird shit lives down there sometimes. When we go to a cenote, we're interrupting a whole ecosystem that's been hidden to us; we had to fucking seek these cenotes out, in the Yucatan, in Slovenia, in Slovakia. And there's millions out there that are unfound. In Mexico I also went to something called a *caleta*, where the cenote meets the ocean, and the salt water and the fresh water meet and then the tide creates a whirlpool right at the shore. It's a little micro-ecosystem within the shore of the beach. Imagine all these rocks almost making an enclosure along the ocean shore, and then within them there is this own little world that's not salty, that's colder and clearer than all the other water, and there's all these birds and fish–it's unbelievable. Chef Éric Werner from Hartwood introduced us to these Mexican dudes who bring him fish; they took us on out to the *caleta* on the boat, where we were drinking Modelo Negras, just chilling. It's just another universe, and when you see it, you feel so appreciative for living.

The Woods. Not heavy-duty hiking, just trekking: doing a little trail, a light hike through the woods up to a rock or a waterfall or a lake or some sort of fresh water that can be jumped into, then walking a little more till you get to a peak or anything looking over something, then enjoying a blunt. Weed just puts you at one with nature, and nature puts you in a state of happiness and fulfillment.

The Vineyard. I have done this literally, lying in the earth between rows of grapevines with a glass of wine, smoking a humongous joint with a lot of fine French hash in it. I took my friend Clovis's hash that he gets from the Arabic men in Paris, the brown shit, and I pressed that out like a dab to make it as pure as possible into a beautiful auburn pungent resin. Also I drove there through the hills of Auvergne in a new sunroofed Mercedes Viano in peanut-butter leather that a sheik usually takes. Crazy consoles. Four huge TVs. The only take me, the sheik, and Usher in this car. Doors open, wine, going nuts. The winemaker Patrick Bouju had given me one of the rarest bottles of his wine called The Basalt, and it flew out of the car–it was such a tragedy. We were wiling out to Metallica, and something flew out of the car. I thought that it was an empty bottle. Then the gendarmes, the state police, pulled us over. The driver held it down, and we continued eating sausage, drinking wine, wiling out. It's an unforgettable moment. We gave the car back–broken bottles, glass, wine everywhere–and he had to pick the sheik up the next day.

The park. The park is where I really learned how to smoke weed, playing handball with Puerto Ricans and different types of human beings. There was always something crazy going down at the park. It gave me a lot in my life–the park is life. You would tell Mommy and Daddy you were going to the park to play, but no, you're going to fucking experiment with drugs and sexual things. You learn about all kinds of things at the park–it's an institution in New York. You learn how to socialize with adults playing ball, you learn how to conduct yourself as a man, how to not cheat at handball–that one was hard for me. If it's near the line, I am calling it a line, 100 percent.

Hawaii's North Shore. It's nice there. You can see every single star. You get a connection to them. You can also lie on a rooftop to feel like you're on the North Shore: Put the wave music on. The stars won't be as intense, but you can get a vibe. I like to put the sound of waves on, or rain, or wolves, or other animals. Hawaii is made of ancient land, formed from the inner core of Earth, you understand? It is what we are. We bust out of a dick, the same way volcanos burst, forming all this new land to lay earth on. I feel like human life is a mixture of dicks, mushrooms, and volcanos: Why are they all a similar shape? They all grow out. Can you explain it any other way?

The street. I always smoke freely in the street, always: I don't care what other people say or if the police stop me. I would be the one who lit up in the street, and everyone would be like, *oh, you're crazy*. I was always that guy, 100 percent, I'll just light the blunt anywhere–I have to feel free. I've only not gotten away with it one time in high school, when I was smoking a blunt by Bayside High School. I've gotten pressed up by cops a bunch of times, but only arrested that one time for weed. It was detectives, they were set up in a minivan with a baby seat, using tricks like they were trying to find a serial killer, all for two kids smoking weed. They bagged us up at nine o'clock in the morning, then we drove around in it for almost seven hours for the rest of their shift–it took almost thirty hours for the whole process, during which they got us McDonald's. (I always get the #2, two cheeseburgers, with no cheese.)

Staircases, hallways, little nooks, rooftops, alleys, and other hidden spots. A big thing for me a few years ago was walking around the city and just finding these little places to smoke. I always loved the hidden spots. Usually we'd meet up around Thirty-Fourth Street and then walk downtown–the momentum was always going toward downtown: Lower East Side, East Village. But mainly we'd just hang out and walk around, see people on the street. We'd literally be walking for hours: You're getting your good exercise, you eat, you chill with people, talk shit, see girls, smoke. That's why there's really nothing like growing up in New York City. We were like mall rats, the people who go to malls all day, except we would just walk the streets all day in New York City and see something different every single moment, every block, every corner, you're still going to see something you've never seen before, which is tremendous. You can walk and smoke and fucking find little nooks and little fucking staircases; it was like finding the illest sample ever, it's like a gem.

The bus. The Q31, coming home from night school. The Q31 was the wildest bus because it would go from Bayside High School all the way to South Jamaica. I was on the football team, so everyone would wile out on the back of the bus, like a school bus. No one would ever pay; we'd all go in the back door. Motherfuckers were literally scared to come to the back of the bus, 'cause no one's going to get left alone on the back of the bus, no matter who you are. The back of the bus was always just a place that you knew you would get tested. *You want to stand in the back with the tough guys, eh?* If it got too crazy, the bus driver would sometimes stop and make everyone get off the back of the bus.

A bathroom. Smoking in bathrooms is a big deal in my life.

3 Musketeers is some next
shit—it's only fluffy nougat.
It's my mom's favorite candy.

Total Fat 6g (9%DV), Sat. Fat 4.5g (23%DV), Trans Fat
Protein 1g, Vitamin A (0%DV), Vitamin C (0%DV), Calc

MILK
CHOCOLATE

Nestlé Raisinets® MILK
CHOCOLATE

21

FROZEN

Raisinets

AND

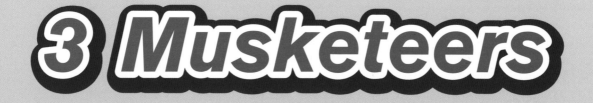

I mean, frozen Raisinets and frozen 3 Musketeers? Holy shit.

22. Losing an Entire Day by Eating Weed

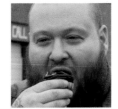

Though I have consumed many edibles*, I prefer smoking–I like the taste of good weed, and I like eating good food. I don't want someone to make me a weed-laced dinner; to me it's a gimmick, like going to Guy Fieri's restaurant on Forty-Second Street. My one famous weed dish is using weed in pasta. I used to do it every morning, with vaporized weed. I was just demolishing myself: This is before edibles and shit like that existed as they do now. I had this contraption called the Volcano; it was like the early vape. It vaporized the weed into this big fucking plastic turkey-brining-bag-looking thing, and then you inhaled the vapor out of the bag. After that, the weed would be vaped, toasty and popcorny and warm. I called it activated.

I used the activated weed to make a fresh tomato sauce for pasta: I'd throw that into some extra virgin olive oil with some fresh baby cherry tomatoes and chiles and garlic and simmer it on low, a beautiful little pasta dish that just happened to have some vaporized weed in there. You can strain it out before you add the garlic and chiles, or you can leave the weed in there, if you like the flavor of weed. If you're using good weed, it's going to taste banging.

And, man, I didn't realize how heavy-fucking-duty it was: The first time I ate it early in the morning, and I don't think I woke up until midday. I passed the fuck out, because I couldn't deal with myself. I was in a corner curled up. I was on the couch, and no one knew what the fuck was going on. I have to smoke a lot of weed to get that feeling. It's hard to obtain that feeling–it's not easy–when your eyes are low and you feel crazy and you're so high, it's a completely different thing.

I made that pasta every morning for a while. I've heard people say that when you cook the weed like that, you can burn it, and it doesn't work, but I've never burned it, and I've always gotten fucked–it's never not worked. This pasta took days off my life: It paralyzes you. You don't really know how hard it is going to hit, so it's kind of a crapshoot every time. I never made cookies–I've made brownies once in a while–but I made that pasta every morning as long as I had that Volcano.

---

* I eat a lot of edibles, especially when flying or being driven long distances, but I try to stay away from edibles that are sugary or have a lot of coconut oil. Everyone makes cake pops, cookies, gummy bears, and brownies, which is, of course, the traditional way to eat weed. Even older people, when they see an edible, it's, what is that, a weed brownie? It's always a weed brownie to older people. Chocolate and sweets cover up the flavor of weed, but I don't mind tasting a little bit of the weed: It's earthy. The weed oil that they use in most edibles is usually called "the clear"; they take a whole bunch of bullshit and strip away everything but the THC with no flavor and just use that. It's oil that you wouldn't sell to smoke; it's just for cooking. I always found that the edible that worked the best for me is not even an edible at all: The last time my guys made a bunch of oil for smoking, they just gave me a big Ball jar filled with it. I would just take a spoonful every once in a while, like a spoonful of medicine.

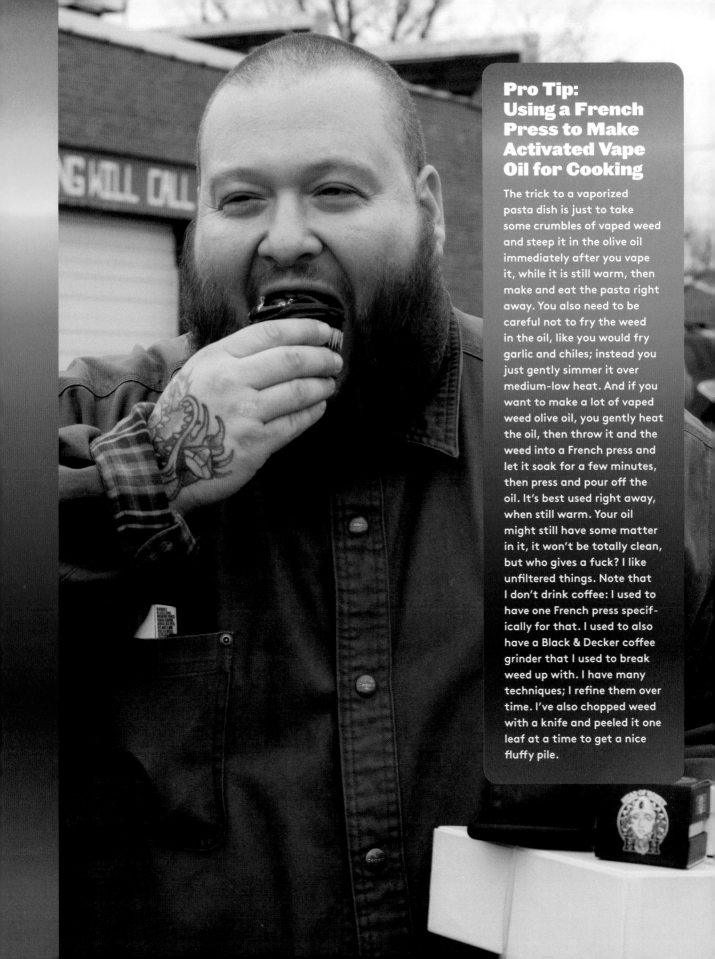

Pro Tip: Using a French Press to Make Activated Vape Oil for Cooking

The trick to a vaporized pasta dish is just to take some crumbles of vaped weed and steep it in the olive oil immediately after you vape it, while it is still warm, then make and eat the pasta right away. You also need to be careful not to fry the weed in the oil, like you would fry garlic and chiles; instead you just gently simmer it over medium-low heat. And if you want to make a lot of vaped weed olive oil, you gently heat the oil, then throw it and the weed into a French press and let it soak for a few minutes, then press and pour off the oil. It's best used right away, when still warm. Your oil might still have some matter in it, it won't be totally clean, but who gives a fuck? I like unfiltered things. Note that I don't drink coffee: I used to have one French press specifically for that. I used to also have a Black & Decker coffee grinder that I used to break weed up with. I have many techniques; I refine them over time. I've also chopped weed with a knife and peeled it one leaf at a time to get a nice fluffy pile.

THE INCR-EDIBLES

MY BOY MIKEY IS A SCHOOL TEACHER. I'VE KNOWN HIM FOREVER— HE COMES OVER TO WATCH SPORTS ALL THE TIME. THE OTHER DAY, WE WERE WATCHING THE FOOTBALL CHAMPIONSHIPS— A WHOLE BUNCH OF US— WE WERE DABBING, DRINKING BEERS...

IT JUST SO HAPPENED I FOUND SOME EDIBLES IN A DRAWER. THEY WERE LIKE 50mg EACH— LITTLE RAINBOW BROWNIE BITES— AND THEY WERE REALLY GOOD. I ATE TWO OF THEM AND I GAVE MIKEY ONE. OH MAN...

FOR SIX HOURS HE WAS IN AND OUT. THE WHOLE TIME HE KEEPS ASKING "WHERE'S MY PHONE?" THAT'S THE QUESTION OF THE NIGHT— BUT HE COULDN'T EVEN GET OUT OF THE CHAIR TO LOOK.

WE WERE ALL CALLING THE PHONE. THERE WERE MAD PIZZA BOXES ON THE TABLE IN THE KITCHEN. WE CLEANED UP— THE PIZZA BOXES GET LIFTED AND IT'S RIGHT THERE THE WHOLE TIME.

LITTLE RAINBOW BROWNIE BITES ™ · FUN SIZE!

I KNOW THAT FEELING, WHEN YOU EAT TOO MANY EDIBLES— YOU'RE JUST FALLING INTO THIS ABYSS...

INTO THIS EVERLASTING NOTHING.

THIS HOLE— THIS DEEP DEEP DEEP HOLE

SOMETIMES I'VE HAD THOSE DREAMS AND I'D WAKE UP ON THE FLOOR.

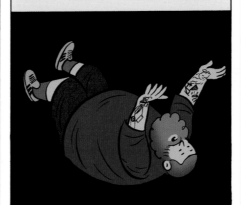

YOU EVER HAVE THAT DREAM WHERE YOU'RE FALLING AND YOU JUST FUCKING FALL OFF THE BED AND WAKE UP?

I USED TO DO THAT ALL THE TIME.

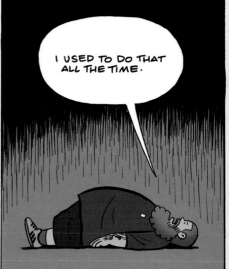

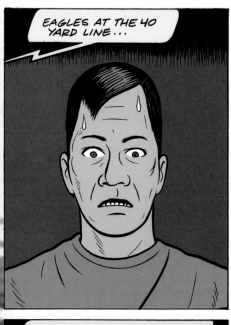

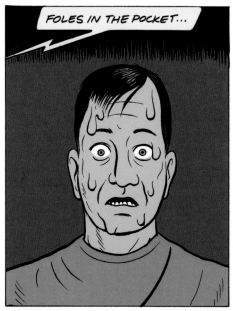

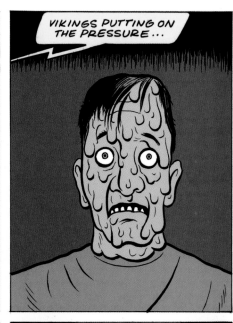

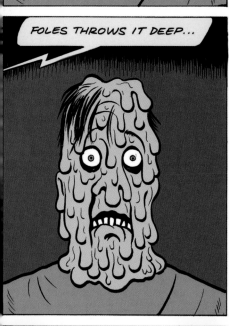

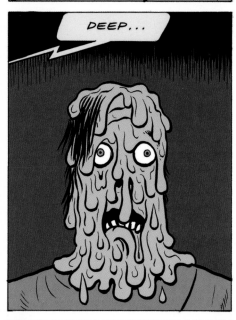

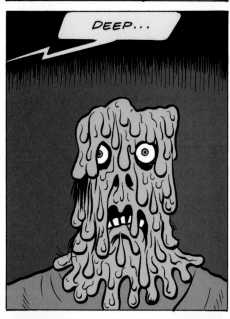

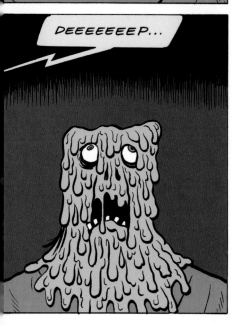

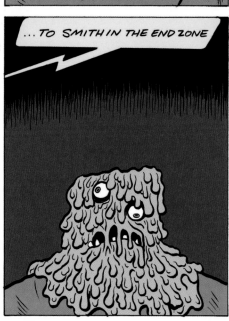

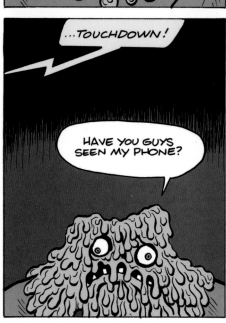

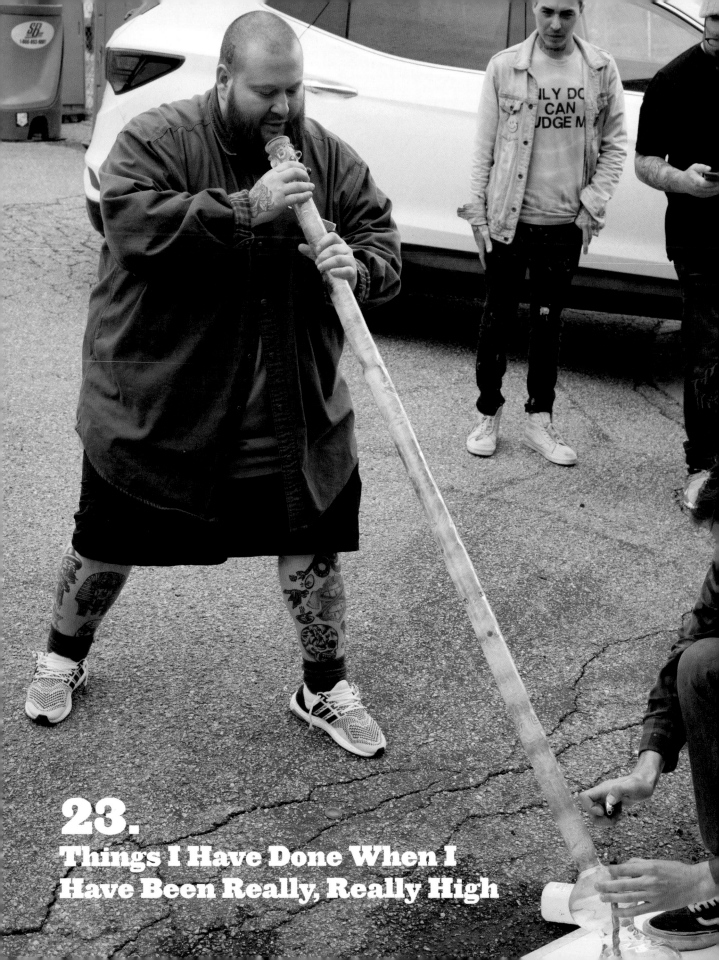

23.
Things I Have Done When I Have Been Really, Really High

1. I haven't gotten on planes.

2. I've made up lies about not being able to make it tonight to stay in to watch reruns of whatever.

3. I have canceled very important shows.

4. I 100 percent bailed on Bono to watch basketball with my girl.

5. I had lunch with my Albanian Uber driver. You wouldn't have that happen to you unless you were a stoner, because you have to be open to the experience. We had Albanian *PITE* and yogurt on a gorgeous sunny day in the backyard of Djerdan Burek in Astoria, Queens.

6. I fell asleep at the dinner table at Capone's with a producer from Def Jam after he got fifteen orders of fried mozzarella. I was new to oil; I was still wet behind the ears. I didn't know what I was doing, and I was fucking trashed. That was way before you could get oil in most places. I'd had some golden yellow piss on paper, gorgeous stuff, buttery, the super bomb from Orange County. I didn't end up working with the producer.

7. I got fully dressed and ready to go out, then passed out in my clothes and woke up in the middle of the night not knowing what the hell happened or where I was.

8. Me, Michael Rapaport, and Body got high in the dressing room while Prince played at a Michael Jordan party. This night was riddled with crazy shit, a series of tripped-out events. All the big athletes—everybody—was there. It was at 23 Wall Street, the twenty-third anniversary of Jordan's shoe. It was incredible, a star-studded night. Some of the greatest athletes who ever lived were in that room, and there were entertainers from all over the place. I was there in shorts. Derek Jeter was there: Me and Jeter embraced for minutes, mad minutes. A few years ago, when Jeter retired, I was in a Jeter commercial, so Jeter fucking showed mad love. I grew up watching him, every single game. You know when you want to meet your idol, and you expect them to be an idol, and then he was, a total gentleman, a total star. Made me feel warm and shit; I walked away in tears. I got Jeter's shoes; I'll never wear them—I'll keep them forever.

9. Moses Malone was there: He was the first person to ever have been drafted to go to the NBA out of high school, straight to the league. He died not long after I met him that day. Magic Johnson was there. And I took a piss in between two of the biggest basketball stars ever: Dominique Wilson and Clyde Drexler. I usually don't like pissing near somebody, but I had no choice.

10. Later we were having dinner, and everyone starts (in high-pitched voice), *OHMIGOD, OHMIGOD*, just screaming, and they start running: Prince is performing in some secret corridor. It was vague; you had to go find him. You literally had to walk out of the building and come back into some other space. It was connected, so you could hear it. So we look for him, we see Prince for a minute, and there were already fucking ten thousand people standing in front of him, you know, so I was like, *AIIGHT*. So me and Michael Rapaport and Big Body were just blowing down in the dressing room. Fucking epic.

11. The moral of the story is, we smoked mad shit, me, Michael Rapaport, and Body. And then Ariana Grande came out to perform at another part of the party in a big hall, and I was just blowing it down right in the room, standing between CC Sabathia, the Yankees pitcher, and Prince Fielder, who was on the Texas Rangers, 'cause they were friends, they lived in the same neighborhood. I had lit up a blunt, a little blunt. And everybody said, *OH, MY GOD!* I always light up a blunt until someone tells you not to. That's my motto: Do it till somebody says stop. Then you say, *OH, I DIDN'T REALIZE*. I'm not a dick about it: It's like medicine to me. You wouldn't be a dick about somebody else taking insulin or fucking pain meds, would you? You can't be a dick about that. And I am who I am. I have a lot of pride about that.

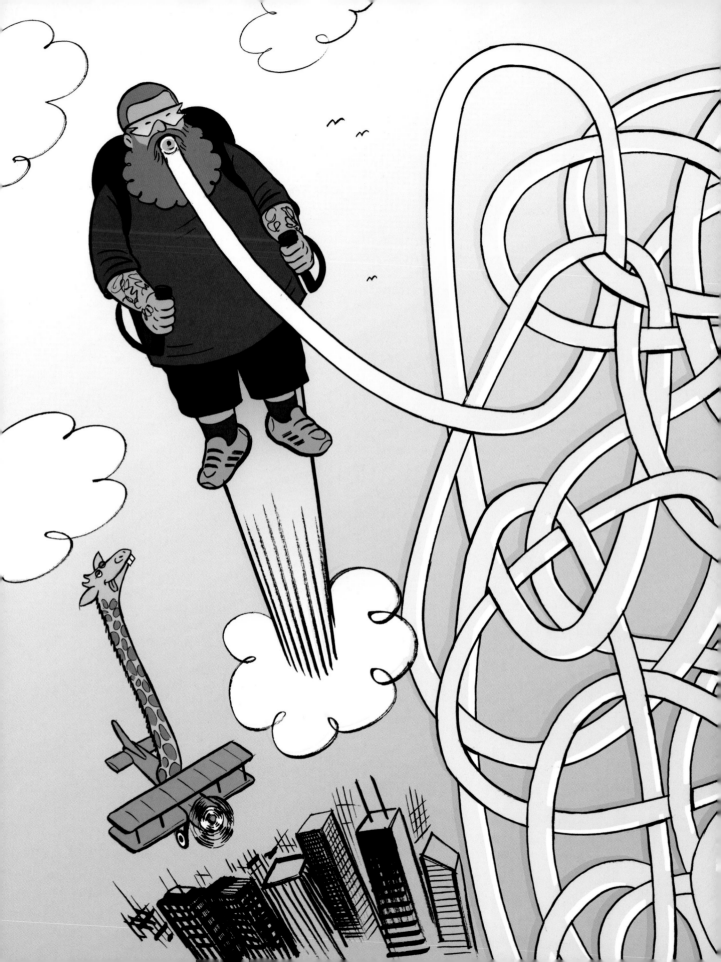

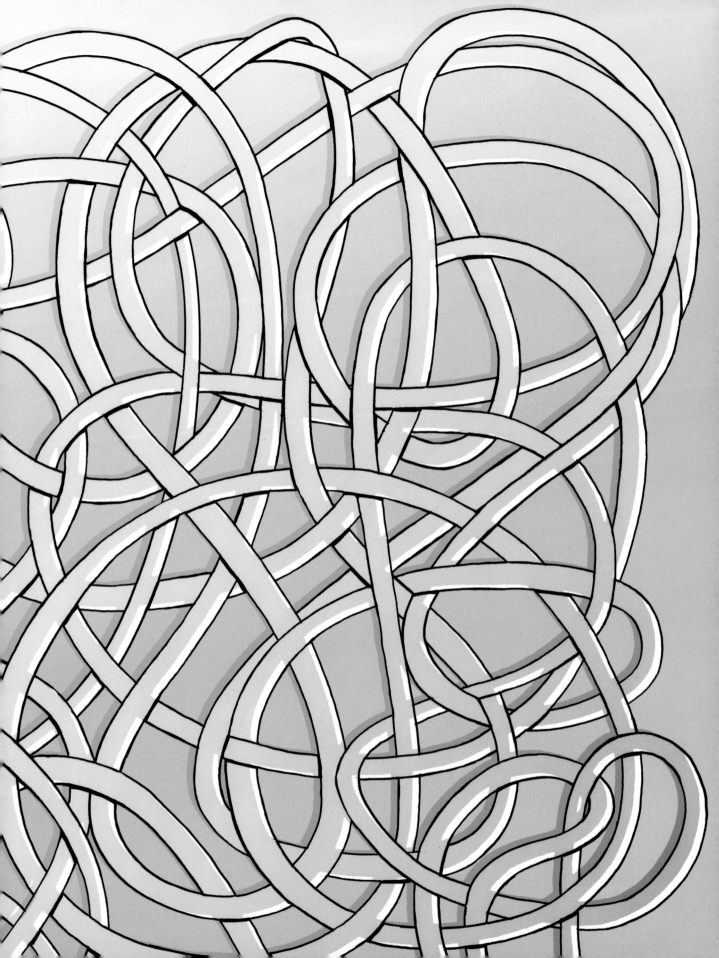

24.

HIGHDEAS
=
Ideas you have
when you're high,
and then it's like
they hit you with the
Men in Black thing.

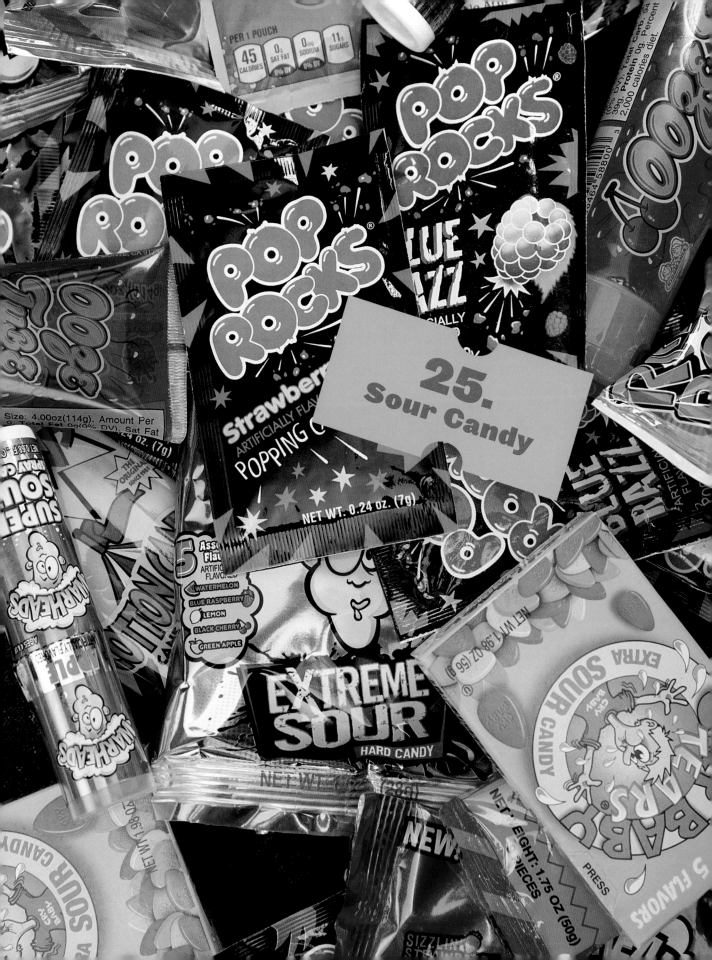

25.
Sour Candy

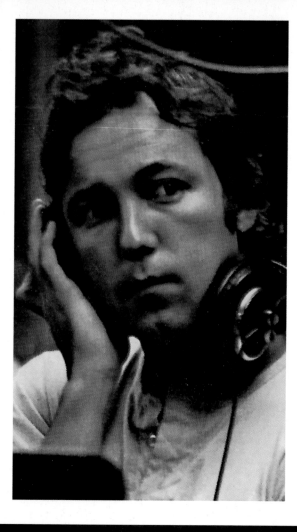

a man and his music

rubén
blades
poeta
del
pueblo

26.
Rubén
Blades

Besides recording the biggest salsa song ever released in any country in Latin America, Rubén Blades is a phenomenal actor, as seen in *The Super* with Joe Pesci. He has played with the Fania All-Stars, one of my favorites, and has a law degree from Harvard. His video for "La Perla" is probably my favorite music video of all time—it's that and "November Rain." There's nothing like seeing live music, even just watching videos of live performances—it's so real, so different from music videos.

27. Sex AND Weed

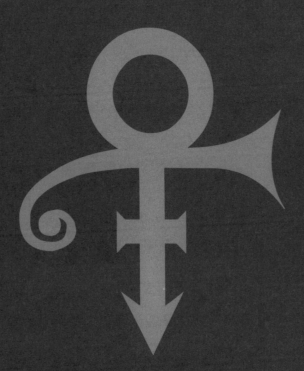

Stoned sex is some of the best sex you'll ever have. It's introspective, it's beautiful, it's poetic, it's musical, it's all of the above. The senses are heightened to another level, you literally feel tingles throughout every part of your body, you have an out-of-body experience where you reach the heavens and you come back down, you see churches and cathedrals and people singing and I don't want to say children dancing, because that's weird, but you know what I mean: all the happy things in life. It just puts you on another wavelength, and if both of you smoke first, then both of you are on the same level; I feel like the weed is a connector. Like your universes have collided and become one. Then, too, it seems to be an aphrodisiac for a lot of people, especially me. I'm just stoned and horny all the time.

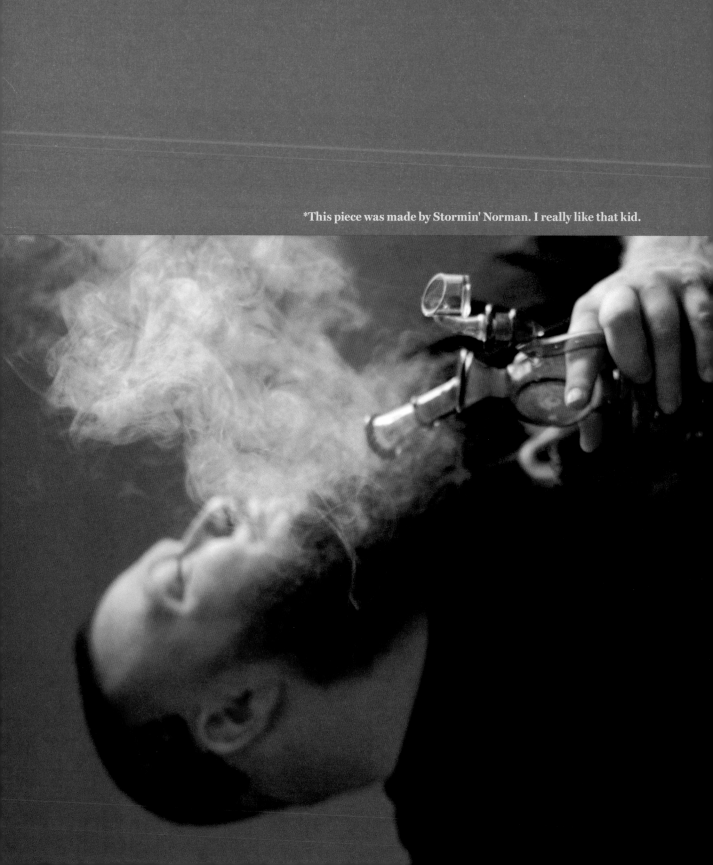

*This piece was made by Stormin' Norman. I really like that kid.

28.
Waking and Baking

This is my morning routine, if you must know: I wake up around 4:59 A.M., though it changes with the sun. At least an hour before sunrise—it's dark for sure. I go and I take a shit for about forty-five minutes; I am on the phone looking at things and shit like that. I get up and go outside on the balcony. I go outside for a little bit. I stretch. Then I come inside, maybe I watch some show, *SportsCenter*, maybe. Maybe I watch *SVU*. Maybe I make pasta, a morning shake, a morning bao with a little A5 Wagyu, a little leftover soujouk. Then after that, my girl wakes up. There's all kinds of crazy commotion as she gets ready for work. At this point I'm hitting the pipe constantly. I definitely smoke before I brush my teeth. It's like the orange juice effect: Toothpaste ruins the taste of weed, I have to drink some seltzer or something. So after I brush I wait . . . seconds. Mere seconds.

I might be able to go back to sleep after a couple of hits from the cup, a couple of tokes from the pipe, but by then I'll sleep on the couch sitting up. Growing up, I've learned how to sleep on planes, sleep in the Uber, get little rests here and there. I can shut my eyes for a second and just restore. These mini-naps are restorative.

And then I go on with my day. My day starts early, and I stay up late. I like to live as much as I possibly can. I don't like to sleep, I don't like to bullshit, I like to live. Plus, there's more hours in the day to get high. I realize that I am literally miserable when I am not high; I'm an asshole to begin with, but I am really an asshole when I am not high. It's like when a cokehead needs his coke. When an alcoholic needs that beverage, when they need that cold one.

Morning Shake

When I was training, lifting weights, I'd have this shake after I worked out. It's just one of those things that taste really good, and you can add protein to it, or Irish moss, or any good fats, or amino acids, or CBD oil.

Serves 2

1 ripe banana, cut into chunks
1 cup (90 g) rolled oats
½ cup (50 g) Marcona almonds
⅓ cup (33 g) cashews, almonds, walnuts, or a mix
1 teaspoon ground cinnamon
1 teaspoon ground nutmeg
3 tablespoons cocoa nibs
¾ cup (180 ml) to 1½ cups (360 ml) unsweetened almond milk
1 to 2 cups (240 to 480 g) ice cubes
Honey to taste

1. Add the banana, the oats, the nuts, spices, cocoa nibs, and ¾ cup (180 ml) almond milk to a blender and process until everything is broken down.

2. Add the ice and a big squeeze of honey and process until everything is smooth, adding more milk as needed or as desired.

3. Taste for honey, adding more as desired, and serve right away.

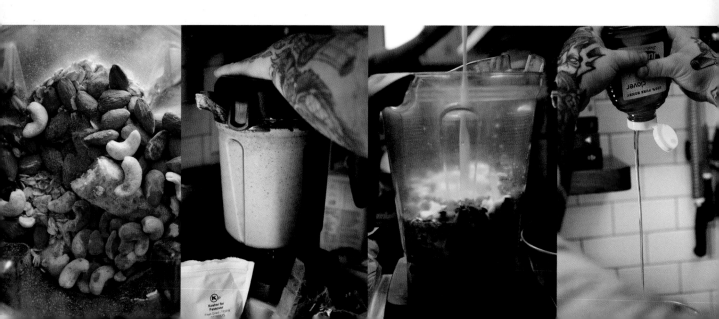

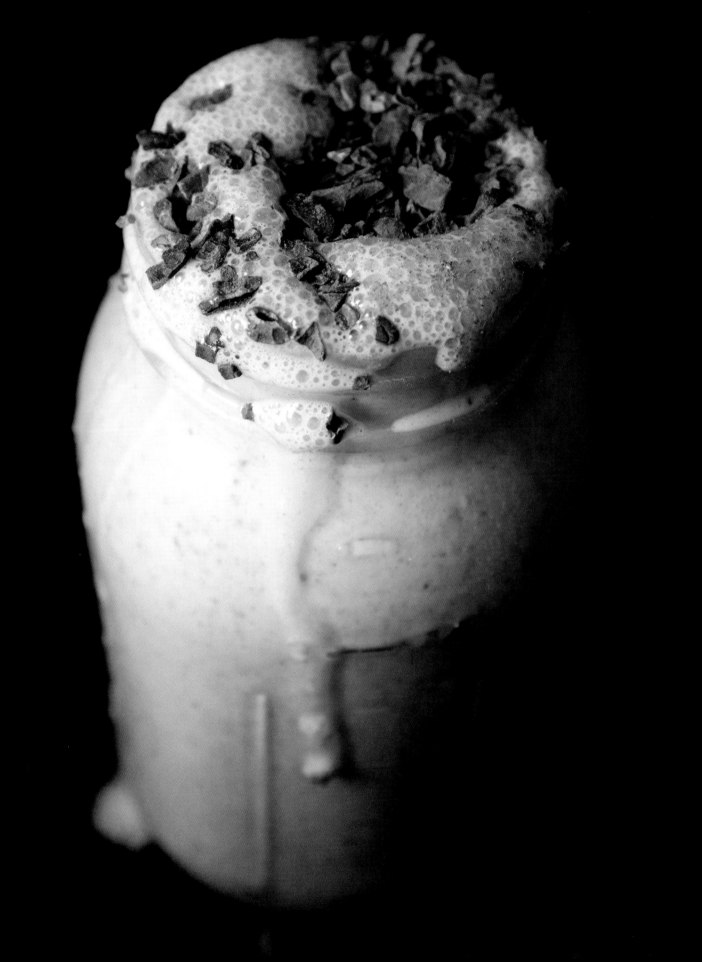

Wagyu A5 Steak

The Wagyu A5 steak is decadent. It's gorgeously marbled. I want to make shoes with that pattern. I had a bunch of it because I had just bought my dog, Coco, $1,000 worth of Japanese A5 from the Japanese beef store on Great Jones Street in Manhattan, just before he passed. Coco ate an entire A5 steak about an inch thick and eight inches long. And he was high off the sour me and him had smoked right before. Then later I made the rest into a breakfast bao, seared on one side, sliced, on steamed buns with cucumbers, scallion, cilantro, and crushed peanuts, with dried garlic and Japanese brown sugar. I go on tangents and buy expensive steak sometimes. I grew up with nothing. It's about $120 a pound, but for this you don't really need that much.

> Note: You can find the bao in Asian markets in the refrigerated section as well as frozen. To warm them just follow the package directions, if you can read them, to steam them. If not, steam them for about 7 to 10 minutes, making sure to check that they aren't getting gummy.

Makes 4 bao

1 (1 pound/455 g) boneless ribeye steak
Kosher salt
Olive oil
4 warm steamed folded Chinese bao, see Note above
1 small Persian cucumber, thinly sliced
1 jalapeño chile, thinly sliced
4 small sprigs cilantro, thick stems removed
2 tablespoons crushed roasted peanuts
2 tablespoons toasted sesame seeds

1. Heat a cast-iron skillet over medium-high heat until it is smoking hot, about 10 minutes.

2. Season the steak generously on both sides with the salt and drizzle on one side with a little oil, then place it oil-side down into the skillet, pressing it down so it is flat against the pan.

3. Let it cook for 3 to 4 minutes without moving it, or until the bottom is black-brown and crunchy. (It will smoke, and that is OK.)

4. Use tongs to flip it over, and let it cook for another 3 to 4 minutes without moving it, or until the other side is black-brown and crunchy.

5. Remove it to a cutting board to rest for at least 10 minutes, then cut it into 1-inch (2.5 cm)-wide slices that should be perfectly medium-rare on the inside.

6. Open the steamed bao and dunk each bun in the juices from the sliced steak on the cutting board. Then fill each one with 3 to 5 pieces of steak, a few slices of cucumber, a few slices of jalapeño, a sprig of cilantro, a dusting of salt, and a sprinkle of peanuts and sesame seeds, if you have them, and eat them soonish, before the buns cool and get crispy on the outside instead of soft and steamy.

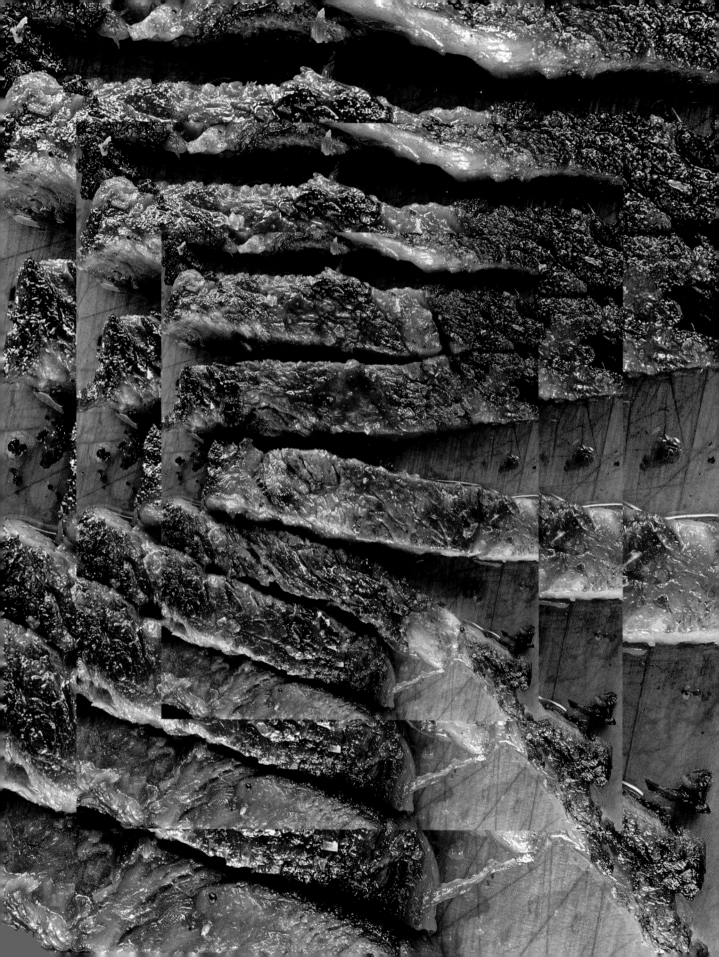

29. Coming Up with New Words for Being Stoned

Schmacked.
Yo, I am fucking
schmacked.

Plastered.

Demolished.

Buffed out.
In a state of
buffamortium.

Flying. *Volando*
("flying" in Spanish).

Loco.

Stupid out of
my mind.

In another
universe.

I'm imprisoned.
I just made that up
right now.

Let the rhythm
hit you.

I can feel the beat
within my heart.
I can feel the love shine
through the dark.*

Ripped, shredded.

Jacked up.

Jacked up off a
shitload of gear.

Final Fantasy 7.

Dunzo.

Crippled.

Smashed.

Devastated.

Bent.

Washed.

Washed up.

Out of my face.

Muffed out.

Toasted, roasted.

Absolutely
astonished.

Fisherman.

Astronaut.

Should have
brought my tap
dancing shoes, like
I was Gregory Hines.

Drugs *got me
speaking Bird.*

* Lisa Lisa and Cult Jam.

30. Five Foods That Have to Be in a Book About Weed

1. Ice cream. I go on lemon sorbet binges too. I love to play with my mind with ice cream: I like tart and sweet and cold together. I like a rich gelato like chocolate or pistachio with the lemon sorbet, so they play against each other. Sometimes I put olive oil on it, too.

2. What were we talking about?

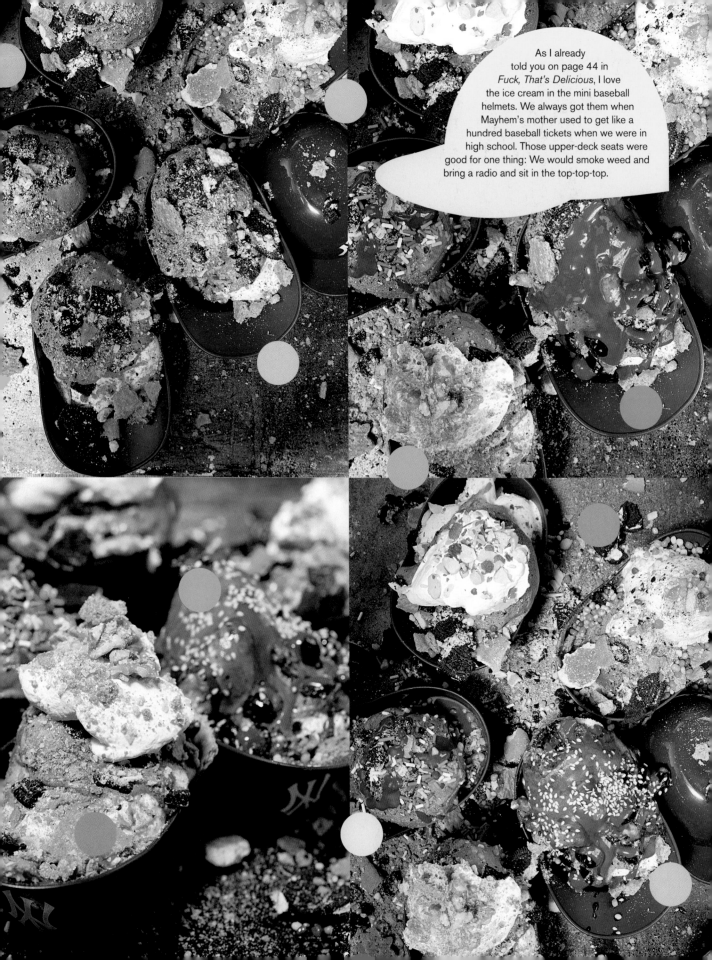

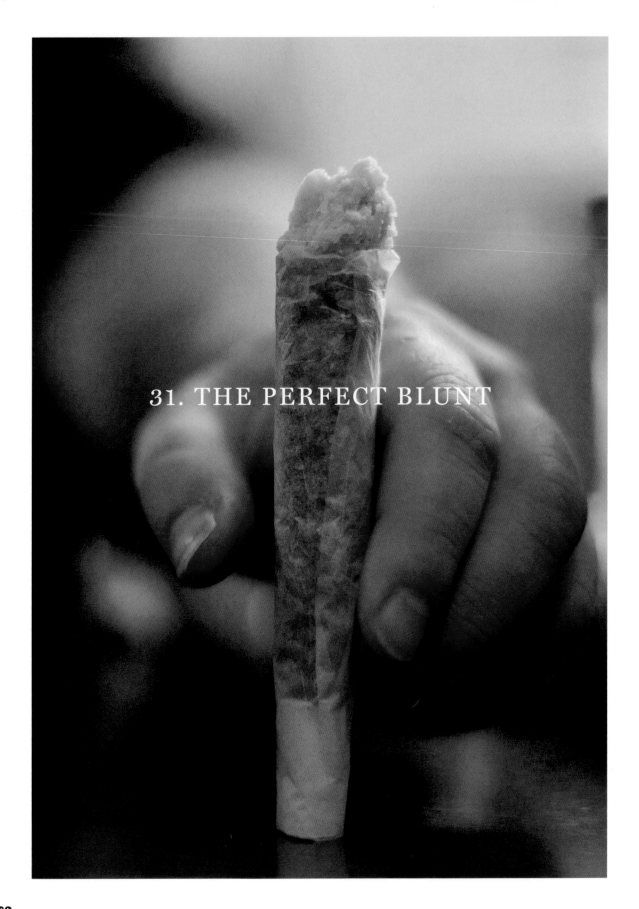

31. THE PERFECT BLUNT

> "The blunt lasted longer than the whole Badu concert.
>
> And when I'm walking back to the whip, I still had a fat clip.
>
> I threw it on the floor and said *shit*.
>
> The whole ride back I ain't say shit."
>
> —from "Chop, Chop, Chop," *Blue Chips 7000*

I'm known as one of the best blunt rollers on the face of the Earth—I'm usually the designated roller. I enjoy rolling blunts: It's just like doing a dumpling. I take half an hour to roll one, because I make sure every piece is broken up by hand, bit by bit. This is kind of like my grandmother picking out the skins of the beans one by one: It's very meticulous. It's like slow food. Three years for the wine. Four years for the cheese. Two hours for the blunt. The goal is to make it look exactly like a cigar again: You could literally take my blunt and you could sell that to somebody, because it's a piece of art. (Some would say that sometimes the mouthpiece was a little tight, but that's just because I like a controlled hit. Some dudes roll it with a humongous mouthpiece, a.k.a. the cannon, so you get a blast. I don't want that.)

I can also roll in any situation: I can roll driving without looking, while standing, while sitting. I used to walk around and have weed in my pocket; if I wanted to roll it, I'd just go into a bathroom, like the one at the twenty-four-hour Turkish spot on the block where Katz's Delicatessen is in Manhattan. You know how many blunts I rolled in there? Oh, man.

I can roll joints too, but I prefer rolling a blunt because it feels good to roll a lot of weed until you have a humongous big-ass cigar. I used to pre-roll five joints every morning. There was a point where I was smoking, like, fifteen of those a day: That's what I did. But you can smoke a blunt longer, anywhere from twenty-five minutes to up to an hour. I have documented how long my blunts have lasted: a whole D'Angelo concert, a whole Erykah Badu concert. One of my favorite experiences was at the Erykah Badu concert. The music was tremendous, and I floated into a zone. I literally had the fattest blunt I could roll, slathered in hash. It lasted an hour and thirty-five minutes, and I still had a clip at the end, when I went outside and threw it on the ground as I walked out to my car. And then I don't think I said anything on the ride home: I was out of my face. It was *Face/Off* time. I was definitely Nic Cage versus Travolta out of my face.

32.
HOW TO ROLL A PERFECT DUTCH

You always need a plastic grocery bag to throw the blunt guts into and a Chinese food menu to roll on, and the freshest blunt possible. I like cleanliness when I'm rolling. Dutch Masters are my cigar of choice because you can roll more, because they're a little larger. I didn't grow up with Swishers, White Owls were nasty, and I smoked strawberry Phillies for a minute, but that shit was disgusting. But for a long time it was always about a vanilla Dutch, so much so that at one point I wanted to get the old Amish-looking dudes from the box tattooed on me.

1. Take off the outside leaf, because it's unnecessary; it's just added tobacco. Some like to roll the entire outside leaf around the blunt, because it makes the blunt last longer, but I've tested it many times with many different people, and the inside leaf always wins: It's thinner and synthetic tobacco.

2. Then you gotta look for the line along this leaf—crack it on the line, where the glue is, and remove the tobacco and discard to the plastic grocery bag. Then there's a piece at the end that's known as the cancer paper. You also have to rip that off: It's helpful to have strong thumbs. I like to unravel the tip a little bit, so that it becomes one big thing. Then you remove the glue: You don't want that. And then you can fit as much weed as you can roll into this paper. And I can roll a lot of weed in this paper.

3. Fill it with weed and roll it up. Boom: A fat blunt. If I want to get crazy, which I often do, I swipe the entire piece up to almost the edge with oil.* I slather it, I mean really apply it heavily.

* Melty weed product of your choosing, such as hash, hash oil, bubble hash, budder, live resin, rosin, or shatter as described in My New Weed Glossary on page 144.

33.
THE RESINATOR

There is a special blunt called the Resinator. The Resinator is the thing. People who got to smoke this blunt were, like, the
chosen few; it was like taking an oath. In the Basement (see "The Hub," page 16),
we would save clips of every blunt we smoked and put them in a jar. Later, somebody would
remove every single clipping of ash, so you only had pure, resinated weed, as in weed that has already
been passed through a blunt, now coated with extra THC.

We would collect thirty or forty of those clips, or as many as there were: Sometimes we would save them for months.
You save them, fill up the jar, then break them up and use the weed to stuff something called a Gotti, because Gotti
always had a big cigar. This was a big cigar of straight-up resin weed, all different kinds of weed, which
we'd proceed to smoke, then barf, then be fucking high out of our mind. The Resinator is a
totally different drug; it's next-level shit. You'd only get to do it once every couple of
months, and then we would save the resin clips from all the Gottis and
roll that again into a special blunt, the extra-extra of the
only good extra. I don't even remember the last
time I kept a clip; now I just throw
them out.

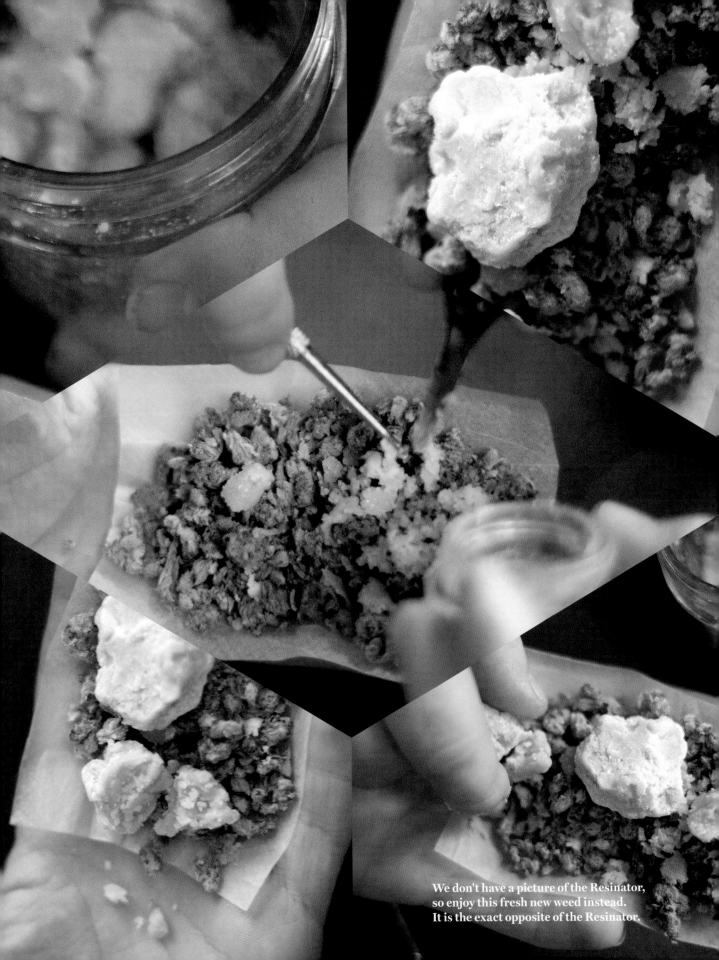

We don't have a picture of the Resinator,
so enjoy this fresh new weed instead.
It is the exact opposite of the Resinator.

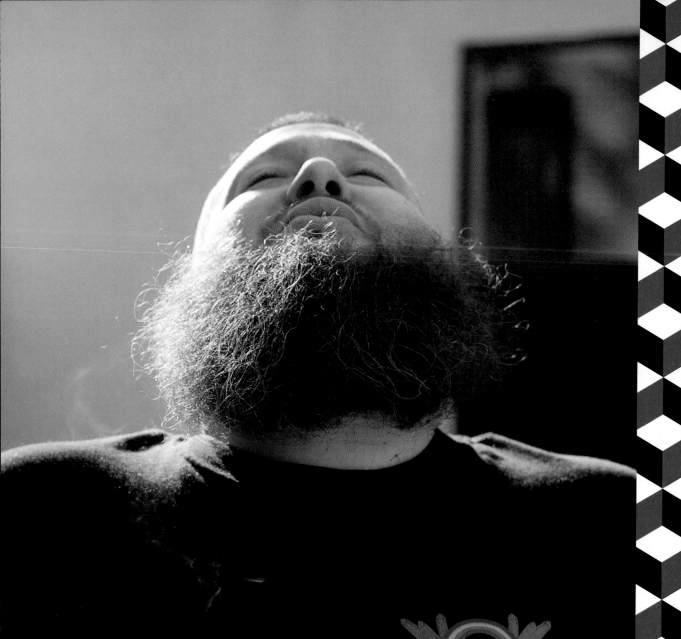

34.

PLAYING CHICAGO

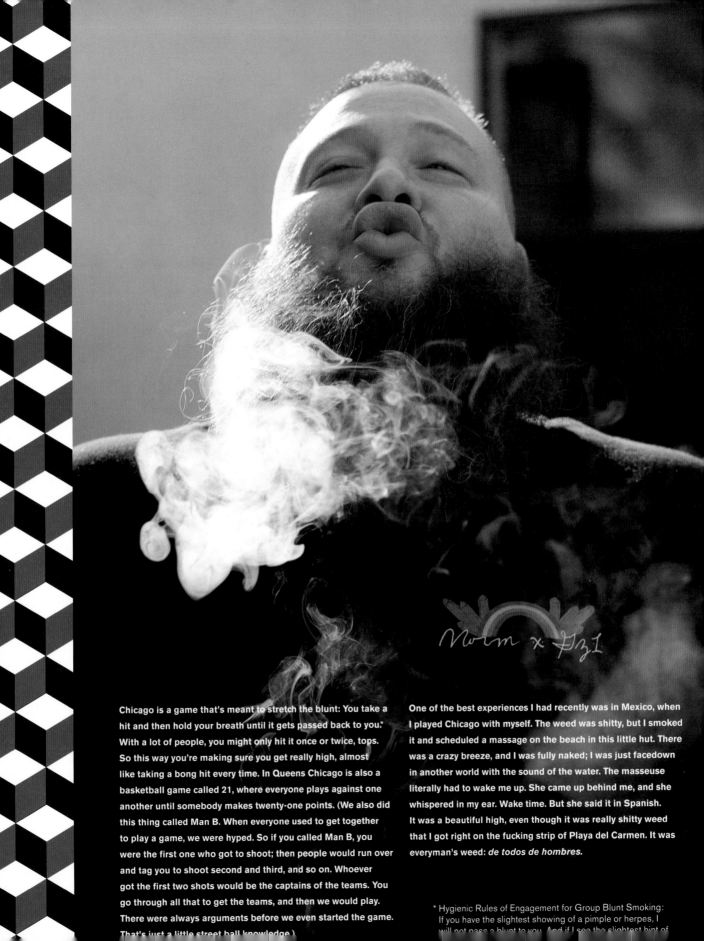

Chicago is a game that's meant to stretch the blunt: You take a hit and then hold your breath until it gets passed back to you.* With a lot of people, you might only hit it once or twice, tops. So this way you're making sure you get really high, almost like taking a bong hit every time. In Queens Chicago is also a basketball game called 21, where everyone plays against one another until somebody makes twenty-one points. (We also did this thing called Man B. When everyone used to get together to play a game, we were hyped. So if you called Man B, you were the first one who got to shoot; then people would run over and tag you to shoot second and third, and so on. Whoever got the first two shots would be the captains of the teams. You go through all that to get the teams, and then we would play. There were always arguments before we even started the game. That's just a little street ball knowledge.)

One of the best experiences I had recently was in Mexico, when I played Chicago with myself. The weed was shitty, but I smoked it and scheduled a massage on the beach in this little hut. There was a crazy breeze, and I was fully naked; I was just facedown in another world with the sound of the water. The masseuse literally had to wake me up. She came up behind me, and she whispered in my ear. Wake time. But she said it in Spanish. It was a beautiful high, even though it was really shitty weed that I got right on the fucking strip of Playa del Carmen. It was everyman's weed: *de todos de hombres.*

* Hygienic Rules of Engagement for Group Blunt Smoking:
If you have the slightest showing of a pimple or herpes, I will not pass a blunt to you. And if I see the slightest hint of

35. Five Foods That Have to Be in a Book About Weed

1. Ice cream. I go on lemon sorbet binges, too. I love to play with my mind with ice cream: I like tart and sweet and cold together. I like a rich gelato like chocolate or pistachio with the lemon sorbet, so they play against each other. Sometimes I put olive oil on it, too.

2. Cereal. And when you're high, it's best out of a plastic cup. I can eat an entire box of cereal from a plastic cup—that's, like, fifteen plastic cups of cereal. I just keep refilling my cup. Cereal tastes better from a plastic cup because of the narrow shape of the cup: It soaks slowly. Also, why do they make the inside bag so crinkly? I get caught eating it at three in the morning.*

3. Pizza.

4. Take-out Chinese food. Chinese places know what to do: They put a lot of Madison Square Garden in there. You can tell when they don't put it in there, 'cause the food doesn't have that shine, that sheen, that taste, that everlasting deliciousness, you know what I mean?

5. What was I thinking, five things? It's everything—all foods have to be in a book about weed. I sold myself short.

* One morning when I couldn't sleep, I poured out an entire box of Lucky Charms cereal onto the table. I removed every single marshmallow, and then I put the cereal back in the box. I love that marshmallow texture—it freaks me out. When my lady went to eat the cereal that next morning, she threw the whole box at me, screaming, why did you do this, you fucking asshole?! But I was stoned out of my mind, so what am I gonna do? So I was looking for something quick and sweet, a quick fix to the pain. Then I just went in. She's the one who could eat the whole box. She's very slim. It takes a lot for her to gain weight, you know? But for me, I could eat one piece of bread (see "Bread," page 200), and it's over for the rest of my life.

This is Alchemist's little area.

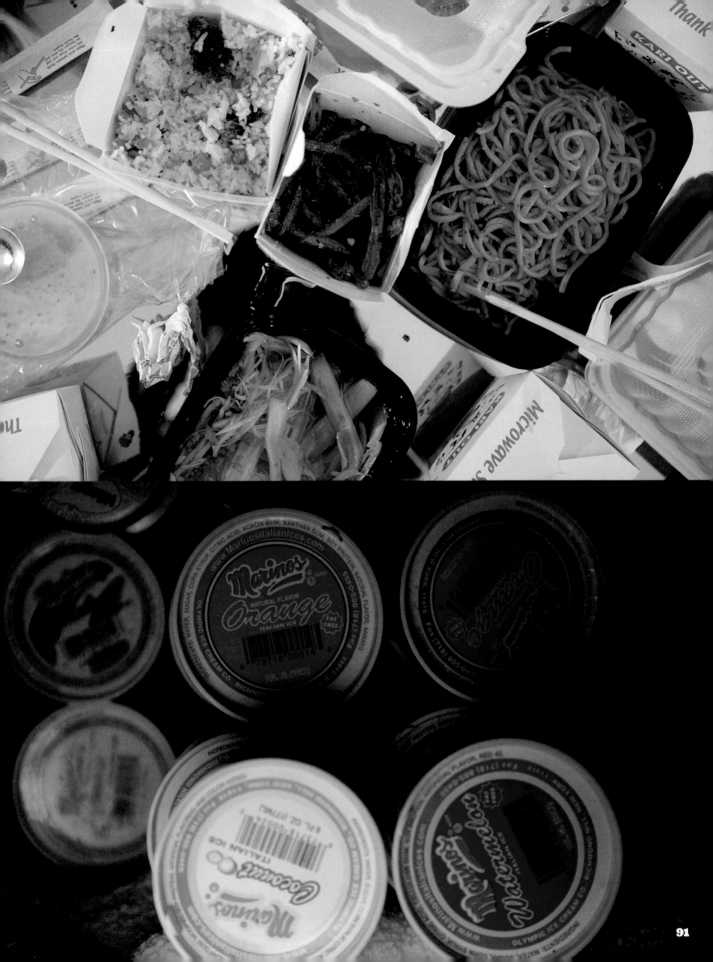

36. Fried Rice

You make this with the rice left over from #4 on page 90, but I make all kinds of fried rice all kinds of ways, from any leftover rice. Like leftover Mexican yellow rice with the little carrots and peas—making fried rice with any yellow rice is lit—or the long basmati Indian rice, or the Caribbean rice and peas made with coconut milk. Oh my god, hit it with a little leftover jerk chicken and sauce? That would be dope. It just has to be leftover and a little dry, not fresh. This should be *easy*—so if you don't have Aleppo chili powder or sesame seeds or fried garlic, dust it with whatever you do have, like something else fried, any type of nut or seed, some good paprika or another chili powder, maybe a little stir-together of rock sugar and crushed peanuts. If you want to get really fancy, cut up the whites of the scallions into long strips for the garnish, the way they do in Chinese restaurants.

Serves 2

5 garlic cloves, smashed with the side of a knife
1 small jalapeño chile, thinly sliced
Kosher salt to taste
2 tablespoons olive or vegetable oil
1 to 2 small hot dried red chiles, crushed, or 1 teaspoon red chile flakes
2 to 3 cups (200 to 300 g) leftover rice
2 scallions, thinly sliced
1 tablespoon soy sauce, plus more to taste
2 teaspoons sesame oil, plus more to taste
1 small handful picked cilantro leaves
1 tablespoon toasted sesame seeds
1 tablespoon fried garlic chips
1 teaspoon Aleppo chili powder

1. Chop the garlic and about half of the jalapeño slices together on a cutting board with a sprinkle of kosher salt until they are finely minced and mashed together.

2. Now remember, this is gonna go down quick: Heat the oil in a medium skillet over medium-high heat until it is smoking hot.

3. Add the garlic mix to the pan and cook, stirring constantly, until it just begins to brown, usually in less than a minute. (Take the pan off the heat for a moment and reduce the heat just a little bit if things start to burn.)

4. Add the dried chiles to the pan, stirring for a few seconds so they are mixed in, then add the rice, stirring and breaking it up with your spoon or spatula as you add it so that every grain is coated in the oil and chile and garlic.

5. Add about half of the sliced scallions to the pan and let them just wilt for a few seconds, tossing and stirring them the whole time. Sprinkle the soy sauce over the top, tossing and cooking and stirring until it is mixed in.

6. Stir in the sesame oil and then add the cilantro, the rest of the sliced jalapeño, and the scallions right at the end, stirring just until the cilantro has wilted. Taste for soy sauce and sesame oil and salt, adding more as desired.

7. Dust the top of the rice with the sesame seeds, fried garlic, and Aleppo chili powder and whatever else you want: extra cilantro, extra scallions, rose petals, candy sprinkles—go crazy.

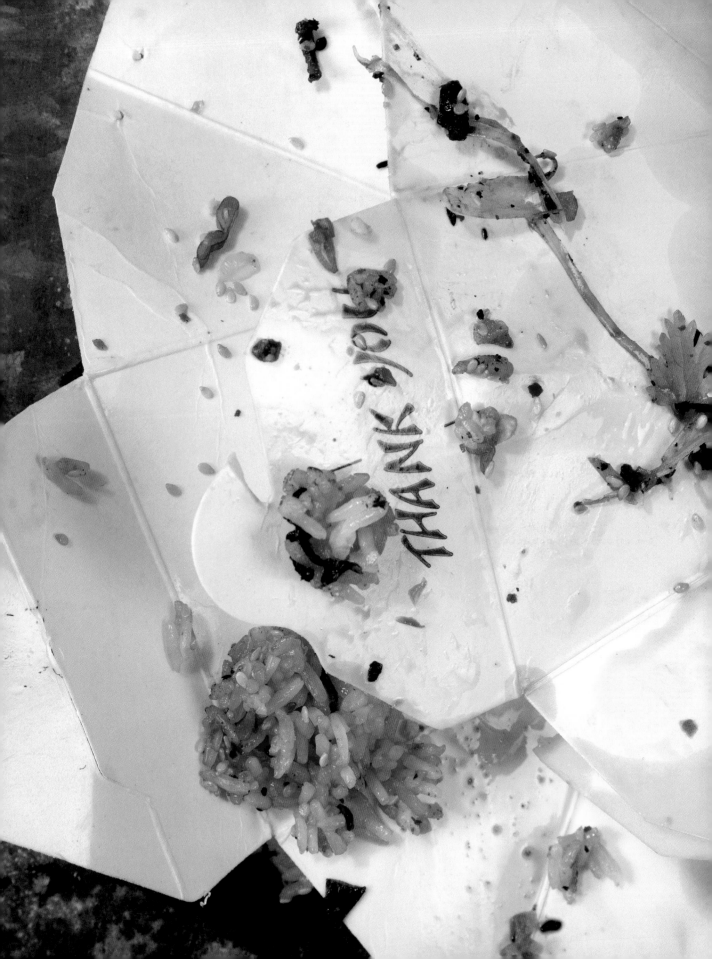

Six More Foods That Definitely Have to Be in My Book About Weed

37. Shawarma

Mad layers of amazing-ness packaged so that you can deliver it directly to your face. And all kinds of condiments that you can put on it, that you can personalize and make it your shawarma. Every bite can be different—that's a stoner move. Everything I do is a stoner move. Everything has to be fucking seventeen plates of different things, even when it's only me. Every time I order a meal, I get what would be considered a stoner move. When I cook, I am stoned, so that's a stoner move too. Though sometimes you just fry a piece of cheese in the pan, and that's that.

38. Korean Barbecue

First off, it's interactive. Anything that's got fire and shit that you do for yourself is next-level: It's, like, whoa. You can do it to your liking, and there's so many different things to play around with, it's almost a toy store on the table.

39. Slush Puppies

You used to be able to go to the store and get your own thing. You pull the lever down, and it gives you just ice and water–type slush, then you squirt your flavor into your shit. It had the dog logo. We used to OD: We'd add every fucking flavor, and they used to only let you get four or five squirts, but I used to get ten squirts from the one on Queens Boulevard. My favorite flavor was all of them, mixed. Green, purple, red, blue. It would turn your mouth a crazy color afterward, and you would drink it so fast, it would give you a brain freeze, like sniffing a fucking rail, I would imagine. Who thinks putting anything that color in your body is good for you? But if they approve it, fuck it. It's like Fun Dip—that's crazed, that shit. Used to unroll the packet, all the different fucking sugars. Just pouring tangy sweet sugar down your mouth.

40. Galaktoboureko

Greek sweet cream cheese custard in phyllo dough covered in sweet syrup, like a cheese-stuffed baklava. You say it like galatikakakako. Even the name is heady. It's the only thing they serve for dessert at Taverna Kyclades in New York; no matter how full you are, it's one of those things you have to have. It is crispy outside, luscious inside, topped with the same syrup

41. Zeppoles

Let me tell you something, my man Pete who lives in my mom's building, yo, he makes the best zeppoles in the entire world in my opinion. They're not overly doughy and fat—he makes them in weird shapes so they get crunchy here and there. He has something wrong with his left arm: His right arm is regular, and I don't know what's wrong with the other arm, but it's smaller and thinner. But it can be used for the perfect motion of making a zeppole and putting it in the oil.

42. Teriyaki Burger

From Tokyo Teriyaki, this Japanese spot in Forest Hills I used to go to all the time, down the alley next to a garage with outdoor seating on Astroturf. I went to junior high school right across the street. An unbelievably delicious burger, a mixture type of spiel, laid into teriyaki sauce on the griddle and allowed to crisp, to glisten. Served on a toasted roll with iceberg lettuce, tomato, and mayo. It was a must. I ate a little bit of the burger, then a little teriyaki, I go back and forth, woo-woo-woo; it's just absolute stoner bliss. Fuck being stoned, you just got to be human, have a heartbeat, a pulse.

43. Capri Sun and String Cheese

Sometimes opposites attract.

44. Being Stoned in School

You would always think that you were covering it up, but the thing is, you weren't. You're late, you're stoned as fuck, probably off some shitty weed, you're laughing, everyone's looking at you. Your eyes are closed. You bake the car out, a Honda Accord, but then you air it out for the last ten minutes, you think that shit's going to work? Then everyone passes around the cologne. The cologne just heightens everything; the teacher is just looking at you like you're a piece of shit, because you smell like a pile of perfumed ashtrays. Everyone starts laughing. There was never even genuine concern from teachers: They were always laughing.

But it was magic: You get that first blunt of the day, you meet up early. Maybe you don't go in right away, you blow it down heavy and then you go to gym, second period. Go play ball, sweaty as a motherfucker for the rest of the day, stinking like weed, 'cause you sweat all that bullshit out of you. Then you leave school again, go drive around a little bit and smoke. Roll one up in the car. Someone always had a bag of weed that was thrown in someone else's lap, and then you rolled it. After I went to Bayside High I went to a school called Outreach in Flushing, where kids have issues. It was a joke: You put all the kids who do crazy shit and bad shit in one place, and now they're doing even crazier shit. By then it was over: There were fights in the lunchroom, people screaming all the time, me cutting every class just to go to lunch every period there was lunch. I had a pass for lunch third, fourth, fifth, and sixth period, I'd leave and come back, or I'd stay and I'd pretend I was the first one there. Then there was this one Eastern European guy who used to watch the door; he always used to try to stop me. Or I always was about walking around with the bathroom pass. There's no way I was sitting in class for the whole time. I would just walk really slowly and just enjoy the hallway. It's always about getting over. I was out of my fucking mind stoned when I took my GED.

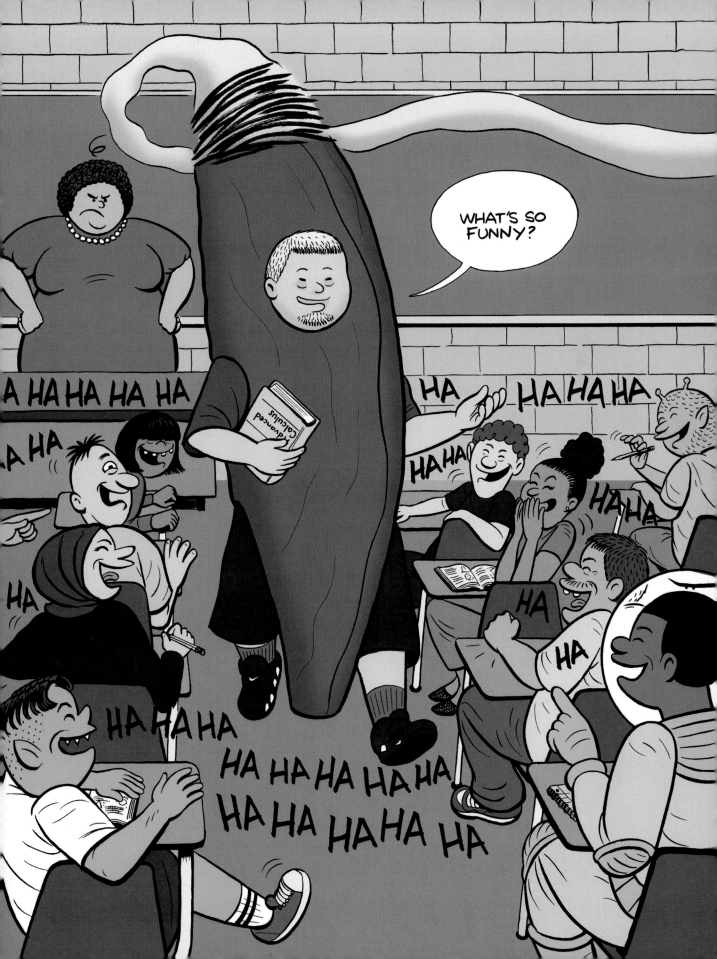

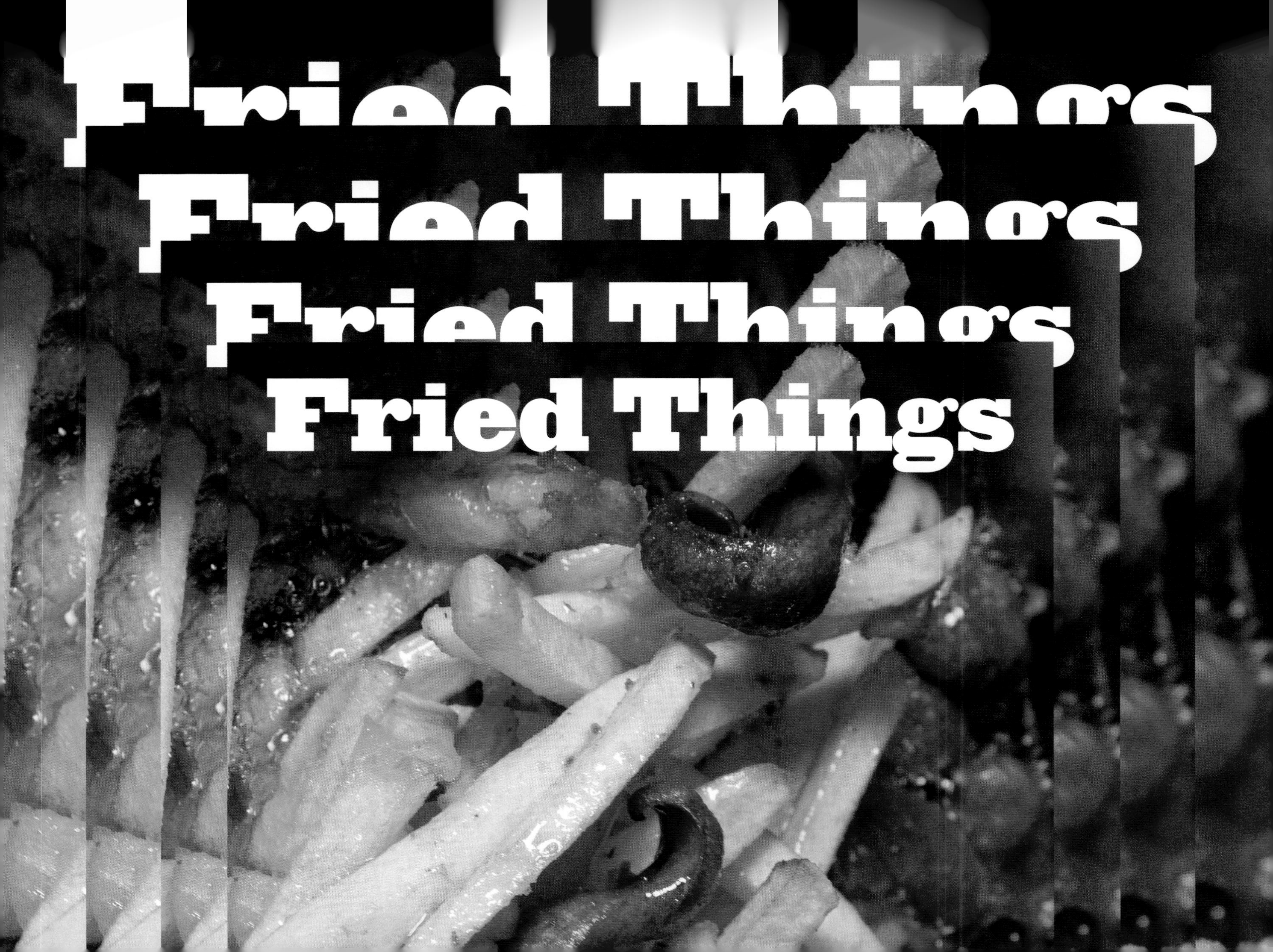

Fried Things

Fried Things

Fried Things

Fried Things

Fried Things
Fried Things
Fried Things
Fried Things
Fried Things

45. FRIED RAVIOLI

I suggest you get the best ravioli you can find—fresh, local. The supermarket kind are last-ditch, but they work too. Cheese ravioli is the go-to, but pumpkin is also very special, though you could use whatever filling you wanted. I like to eat fried ravioli with tomato sauce, like the one I make for the ziti on page 49, but you don't have to—they are good solo, or just a little grated Parm is nice also. Be sure to buy two packs of ravioli and some mozz and make the frittata on page 102 at the same time.

Serves 4

Extra virgin olive oil for frying
3 large eggs, beaten
1 15-ounce (425-g) package plain bread crumbs
Kosher salt to taste
Freshly ground black pepper to taste
1 9-ounce (255-g) package fresh ravioli, any flavor

1. In a large skillet or Dutch oven, heat about 2 inches (5 cm) of olive oil over medium to medium-high heat until it begins to shimmer. Line a small serving bowl or plate with paper towels.

2. While the oil heats, place the eggs in a large mixing bowl and the bread crumbs in a flat cake or baking pan. Season the bread crumbs to taste with salt and pepper.

3. Add the raviolis to the bowl with the beaten eggs* and move them gently about until they are coated, then add them one by one to the pan with the bread crumbs, tossing until each ravioli is coated with bread crumbs.

4. Add the coated ravioli to the hot oil, shaking off any excess bread crumbs, being careful not to crowd the pot. (Cook them in batches if necessary.) Let the ravioli cook for a few minutes until golden brown on both sides, flipping them over from time to time.

5. Remove the ravioli from the pan to the paper-towel-lined bowl or plate and serve hot.

* Save the leftover eggs for the frittata on page 102. Toss the bread crumbs, though.

46. Leftover Ravioli Frittata

This recipe came to be because we were too lazy to make a second batch of fried ravioli, so we just dumped the whole second bag into the leftover eggs and made a frittata. Even though I hate browned eggs, I love to make frittatas. In this frittata—the ravioli crisp up on the top where they poke out of the egg batter and you get a crazy crunch. It has just a little egg, just enough to make everything adhere, so it's almost more like ravioli pie. It's amazing.

Serves 4–6

3 tablespoons extra virgin olive oil, plus extra for drizzling
2 cloves garlic, smashed with the side of a knife and minced
Leftover beaten eggs from making the fried ravioli on page 100, or 2 large eggs, beaten
1 9-ounce (255-g) package fresh ravioli, any flavor
Kosher salt to taste
Freshly ground black pepper to taste
½ cup (62 g) finely grated Parmigiano-Reggiano cheese
4 ¼-inch (6-mm)-thick slices whole milk mozzarella, preferably Polly-O
1 small handful fresh basil leaves roughly torn, optional

1. Preheat your broiler.

2. Heat the olive oil in an oven-safe medium skillet over medium heat. Add the garlic and let it cook just until soft, stirring occasionally, about 3 minutes.

3. While the garlic cooks, combine the beaten eggs and the ravioli in a mixing bowl with a pinch of salt and pepper, tossing so that all the ravioli are coated in the eggs. Add this mixture to the pan with the garlic and remove it from the heat.

4. Cover the top with a fine dusting of Parm—you can just grate it right over, that's what I do—then arrange the slices of mozzarella evenly around the pan.

5. Drizzle the top of the frittata with more olive oil and broil it until the top is golden-brown, about 3 to 5 minutes at most.

6. Slide the frittata onto a cutting board or serving plate, dust the top with the basil leaves and any leftover Parm, and cut it into squares or slices.

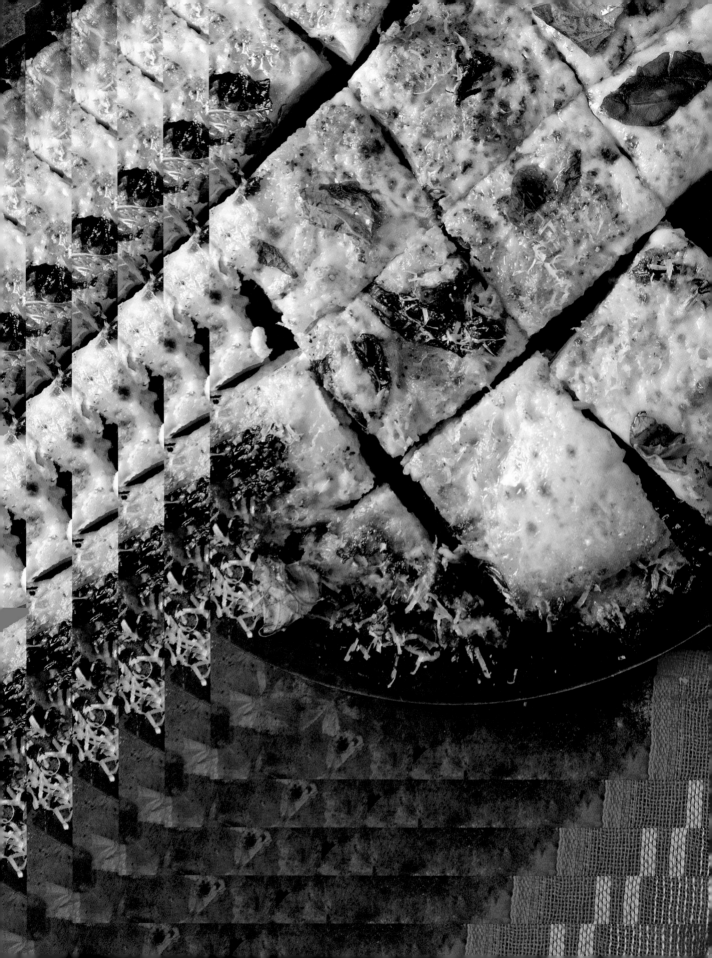

47. Fried Pizza

I could open up a restaurant and sell these, that's how good they are—nobody would ever know it was pizza dough from a can. Before you make this, you must—I mean must—watch Sophia Loren fry pizza in the 1954 black-and-white Italian movie *L'oro di Napoli*, in a scene called "Pizze a Credito." It's on YouTube. You can also top this dough with just about anything you want: Pudding. Ice cream. Whipped cream. Custard cream. Jam. All of the above.

Note: If you can't find stracciatella cheese, which is the little shreds of soft mozzarella mixed with cream found in burrata, which is kind of a form of fresh mozzarella, you could buy burrata and pull out the insides. You could also use fresh mozzarella, if that's all you can find, but it won't be as amazing.

Makes 2–3 pizzas

1 28-ounce (794-g) can plum or San Marzano tomatoes
Extra virgin olive oil
Kosher salt to taste
1 small handful fresh basil leaves
1 13.8-ounce (391-g) tube premade pizza crust
8 ounces (1 cup/226 g) stracciatella, at room temperature (see Note above)
1 cup (124 g) grated Parmigiano-Reggiano cheese

1. Make the sauce: In a mixing bowl, crush the tomatoes with your hands and stir in ½ cup (120 ml) of the olive oil, salt to taste, and the basil, making sure the basil leaves get nice and wilted.

2. In a deep, wide skillet or a Dutch oven, heat about 2 inches (5 cm) of the olive oil over medium to medium-high heat until it begins to shimmer.

3. While the oil heats, pop open the can of dough and unroll it on a clean kitchen counter or cutting board. Use a sharp knife to cut it into 3 or 4 rectangles—essentially you want the pieces to fit comfortably in the skillet with the oil.

4. When the oil is hot, put one of the dough rectangles in the pot and let it fry, flipping it once or twice, until it is golden brown on both sides. This takes only a minute or so, so pay attention.

5. Remove the pizza to a baking sheet, serving tray, or clean cutting board. Use your hands to top the pizza with some of the tomatoes and basil, making sure to drizzle some of the juices over the dough. Dollop on some of the stracciatella, sprinkle on some of the Parm, and drizzle more olive oil over the top. Then cut or tear into it as you please.

6. Repeat steps 4 and 5 above with the remaining dough.

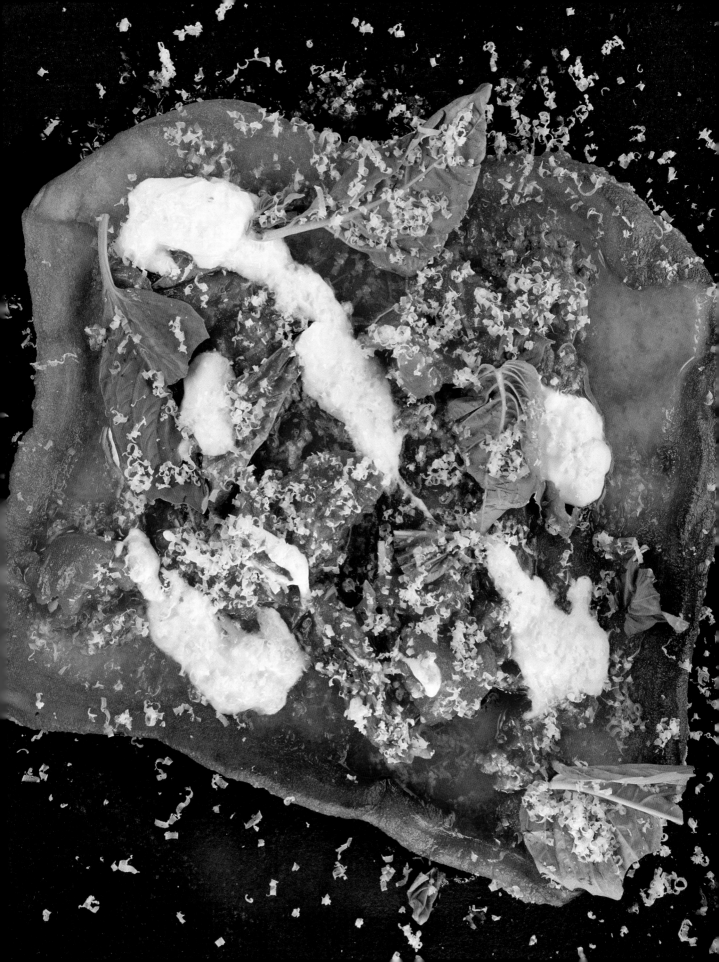

48. Salchipapas

Salchipapas is French fries fried with hot dogs, originally from Peru but now from all over Latin America. What I do when I make any fry is, I pre-fry the potatoes at a lower temperature to blanch them and get them soft, then fry them again at a higher temperature to get them golden brown and crunched. Except in this case you throw the hot dogs in there on the second fry. How could it be bad? The traditional sauce would be pale pink mayo-ketchup, which is exactly what it sounds like, maybe with an added touch of garlic powder.

Note: I prefer a good-quality dog for this dish, something smoked over hickory or applewood, something without too much crap in it, maybe from the local butcher.

Serves 4–6

Canola oil, vegetable oil, or even olive oil, for deep frying
4 Idaho potatoes
4 good-quality hot dogs (see Note above)
Flaky sea salt to taste

1. Fill a mixing bowl with cold water. Peel the potatoes and cut them lengthwise into ½-inch (12 mm)-long fries, placing them in the bowl with the cold water as you go. They don't have to be super clean, they can have a little peel here and there, but I like peeling potatoes.

2. Fill a large Dutch oven about halfway up with the oil and heat it over medium heat, just until the oil begins to move around. It should be a low heat here for the first cook, around 250°F (121°C).

3. Line a baking dish with paper towels. Add the fries to the oil and let them cook until they are soft when pierced with a knife, slightly translucent with a little droopiness, but not really browning yet. It's like you're blanching them in the oil. (You may need to fry them in batches if they don't all fit into the oil at the same time.) When they're done, lift them out with a slotted spatula, place them in the baking dish, and put them into the fridge or freezer to cool.

4. While the potatoes cool, raise the heat under the oil to medium-high, or until it reaches about 350°F (165°C), and line a serving bowl or baking sheet with paper towels. Cut the hot dogs on the bias into 1-inch (2.5-cm) slices, and remove the potatoes from the fridge or freezer.

5. Add the hot dog slices to the hot oil and let them cook for about 20 seconds. (If you had to do the fries in batches, add the hot dogs in batches too, because they have to be fried together—that's the whole point.)

6. Add the fries to the hot oil with the hot dogs and let everything cook—stirring with a slotted spoon or strainer—until the hot dogs curl up and brown on the edges and the fries are golden brown and crispy. If the hot dogs are way done and the fries aren't yet crispy, it's okay—they'll be good just cooked through and soft too.

7. Strain everything to the paper-towel-lined thing you prepared, dust the fries with a little salt, and serve with a sauce of your choosing or your creation.

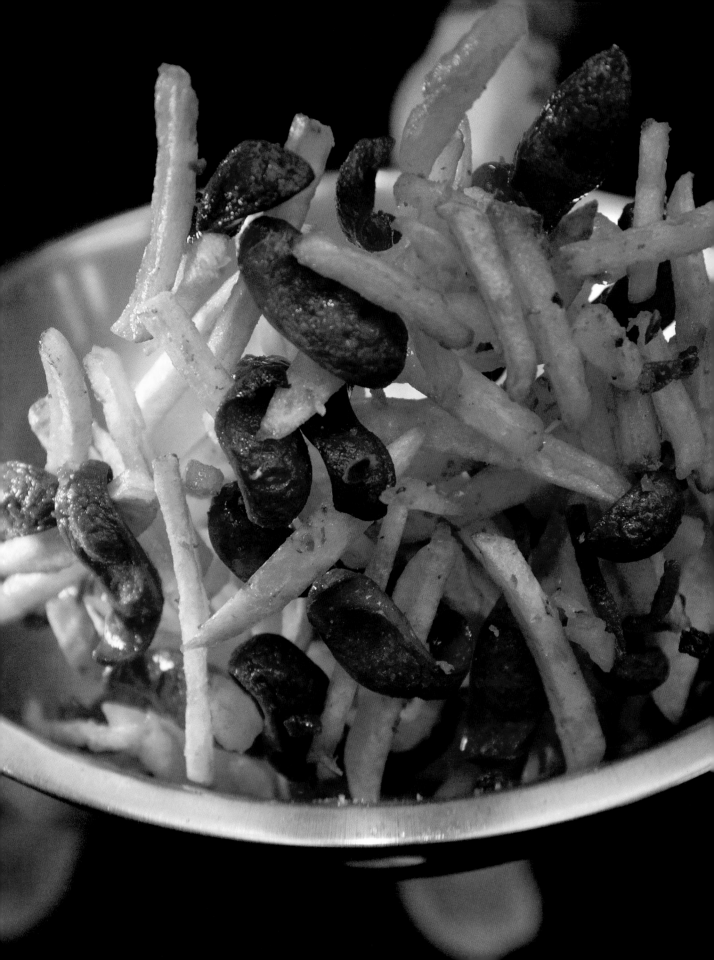

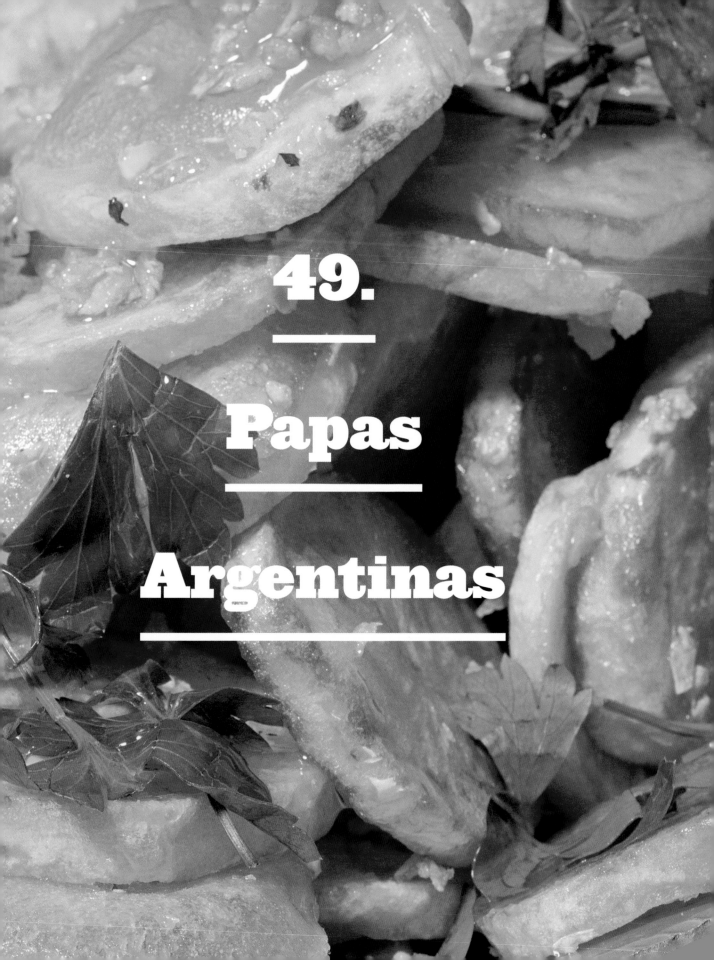

49.
—

Papas
———

Argentinas
———

This is the way my mom used to do these when she was making steak and potatoes. Instead of frying the potatoes once low and twice high, she would leave them in the oil and slowly turn the heat up, so they would get almost empty on the inside, delicate, mashed potatoesque, and fluffy— a really gorgeous puff. There's no more bullshit carb left in there. I top them the way the Argentineans do, with lots of fried garlic and torn parsley.

Serves 4–6

Canola oil, vegetable oil, or even olive oil, for deep frying
1 head garlic, peeled and minced
4 Idaho potatoes
Flaky sea salt to taste
1 small handful fresh parsley leaves

1. Heat 2 tablespoons (30 ml) of the oil in a medium skillet over medium high heat. Add the garlic and cook it until it is golden-brown and almost crispy, about 5 minutes, being careful not to let it burn. Remove the garlic to a plate or bowl and set it aside.

2. Fill a mixing bowl with cold water. Peel the potatoes and cut them crosswise into ½-inch (12 mm)-thick coins, placing them in the bowl with the cold water as you go.

3. Fill a large Dutch oven about halfway up with the oil, and heat it over medium heat to 250°F (121°C) or just until the oil begins to move around.

4. Place a cooling rack in a baking sheet. Add the potato coins to the hot oil, making sure not to crowd the pan. (You may need to do this step in batches.) They will lower the heat slightly; once the oil has reached 250°F (121°C) again, raise the heat slightly so that the oil is at 300°F (149°C), or shimmering slightly. Let the potatoes cook for 10 minutes, then raise the heat again so that the potatoes are cooking at a full bubbling fry, or 350°F (175°C). Let the potatoes cook until they are a dark golden brown and puffy, with no moisture left inside of most of them, then remove them to the rack set in a sheet pan.

5. When all the potatoes have been removed from the oil, transfer them to a serving bowl, sprinkle them with sea salt and the fried garlic, and tear the parsley leaves over the top.

50. Fried Cheese, Fried Salami, and Tostones with Aji

At home I like to take soft white queso de freir—literally, frying cheese—take a nice piece of that and throw it in the deep fryer or a bunch of oil. Aha ha ha. It gets all crunchy and fucking crispy on the outside and then soft and fucking salty gooey on the inside; it's fucking next level. I started doing that working in kitchens with Dominicans. They do it with fried salami and mangu (boiled green plantains) for breakfast, but I do the plantains sliced, fried, and smashed as tostones, which is also the base for mofongo. Like French fries, you must fry tostones twice: one time to soften them, and one time to make them hard again. And you must serve them with aji, or garlic sauce made with a shitload—I mean a real fuckload—of fresh garlic.

Serves 2

2 green plantains
Olive oil
Flaky sea salt to taste
4 ½-inch (12 mm) slices Dominican or Jewish salami
4 ½-inch (12 mm) slices queso de freir
Aji, recipe follows

1. Peel the green plantains. It's not the easiest thing in the world to peel these; you have to cut off the ends of the banana and make three long scores lengthwise in the skin of the plantain, then peel it away.

2. Cut the green bananas into 2-inch (5 cm) chunks.

3. In a deep skillet or Dutch oven, heat about 2 inches (5 cm) of olive oil over medium heat until it begins to move around in the pan, about 275°F (135°C). Set a cooling rack into a baking sheet.

4. Fry the plantains—a few at a time if necessary—until they have softened but not browned, about 3 to 5 minutes. Remove them from the pan to a cutting board.

5. This next part is fun: Smash them down with a coffee mug or wooden mallet or the side of a cleaver. It's OK if they get a little funky; I like things a little funky.

6. Increase the heat to medium high so that the oil is about 350°F (175°C) and fry the plantains a second time for about 3 to 5 minutes until golden brown and crackly around the edges.

7. Remove them to the rack set into a baking sheet, and sprinkle them with flaky sea salt. Keep them warm while you fry the cheese and salami.

8. Heat a drizzle or two of olive oil in a medium skillet over medium-high heat. Add the salami slices and let them fry for a minute or two on both sides until they are dark brown and crispy on the edges. Remove the salami to a serving plate or bowl, and add a little more oil to the skillet if it is dry.

9. Put the slices of cheese in the skillet and let them fry for a minute or two on both sides until they are heavily browned and crispy on the edges and gooey on the inside.

10. Put the fried cheese on the serving platter or in a bowl and serve it with the fried salami, the tostones, and aji.

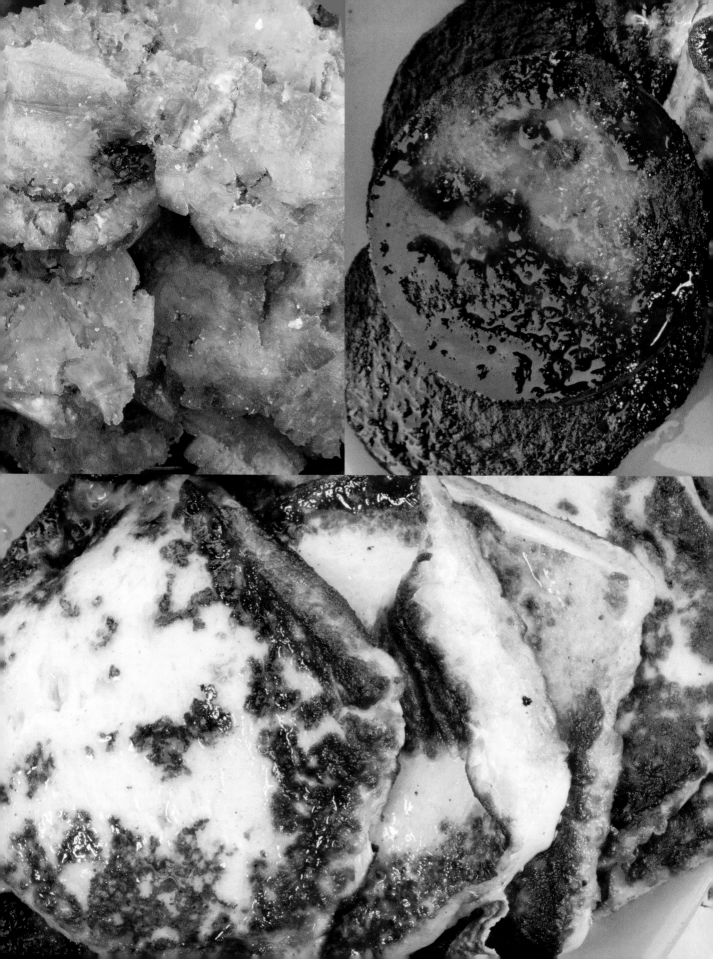

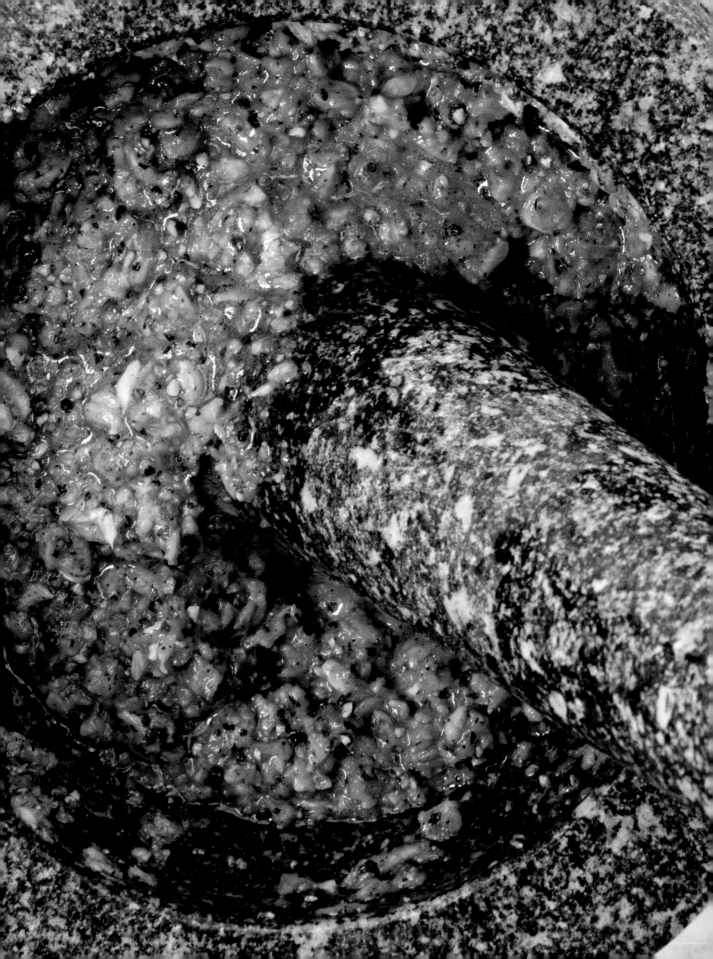

AJI

The mixture of vinegar or lemon juice with the oil gives this a nice smoothness—I use extra virgin because I like the flavor, so with me you also get the flavor of olive oil in this sauce. Use it if you like it. This is called many things—mojo de ajo, mojito—whatever the fuck you call it, it's always a mashed-up garlic thing.

Makes about 1 cup

1 cup (135 g) garlic cloves
¼ cup (40 g) whole black peppercorns
Sea salt to taste
Juice of 2 lemons or 2 tablespoons white vinegar, plus more to taste
Olive oil or vegetable oil
White vinegar, to taste

1. Crush the garlic and peppercorns with 2 pinches of salt with a mortar and pestle until it forms a good paste. (You can also use a food processor or a blender.)

2. Add the lemon juice, mashing until it is well incorporated, and then slowly add oil one spoonful at a time, crushing and mashing after each addition. When the mixture is smooth and the consistency of salsa verde, taste for salt and lemon juice/vinegar, adding more as you like.

3. This will last for 2 days in the refrigerator but should be served at room temperature.

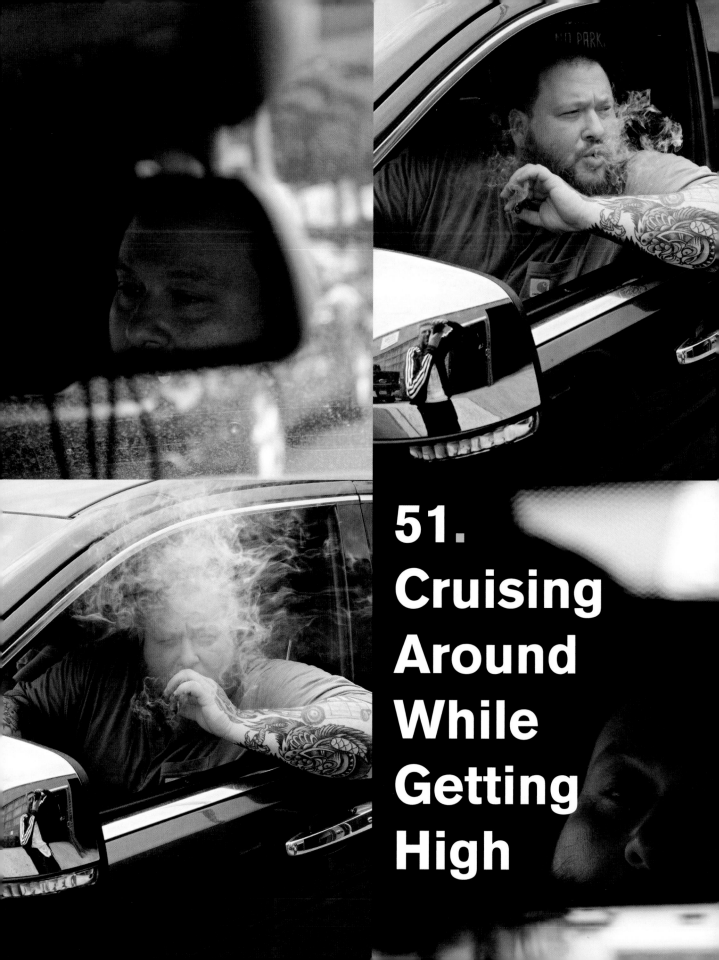

51.
Cruising Around While Getting High

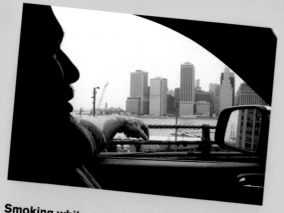

Smoking while cruising is ill. You are doing two things at once that both give you the feeling of real freedom: driving and getting high. Riding around while getting high is pretty much one of my favorite things to do, to this day. It's like a video game of life. Maybe early on it started because we couldn't smoke the weed at home, so we'd have to get in the car to smoke, but eventually it turned into a joy thing, at any age.

Back in the day, my friends and I had a smoke driving tour that we would go on almost every day, multiple times a day: We would get into my car and go out to many different highways where you would never have to stop or get off, like the Belt Parkway or the Cross Bronx or the Long Island Expressway. (If you got on the Jackie Robinson Parkway in Queens, which is a nice drive, you would have to finish the blunt by the time the road exited at Pennsylvania Avenue in Brooklyn, which is a hot block. At nighttime, seven out of ten times, you get pulled on Pennsylvania Avenue.) For years I'd try to always make sure I was in the car on one of these routes between 10 A.M. and 1 P.M., so I could cruise around stoned listening to sports talk radio, when Evan Roberts and Joe Benigno came on at midday.

With a smoke driving tour, what you really want is continuous movement, because it's nice to cruise: You listen to music, and it's like you're on a rolling couch, literally a rolling chill situation. To me, Cadillacs are the best cars to smoke in, because they're truly like rolling couches. I used to have a beautiful Cadillac, a '97 DeVille. Champagne, with white-wall tires. I bought it at auction for seven grand, with only thirty thousand miles on it.

But the day I brought it home, it fucking overheated on me in Harlem. The engine seized. I had to buy a brand-new engine for three grand. It took three months to get it back on the road, and it was never the same. I'd bought a lemon. It's because the engine block is aluminum: When it gets too hot, it melts. I had it for six months: I used to cruise around blasting rap music, smoking stupid weed by myself. I would have the seat so far back that it literally looked as if there was no one driving the car. I'd pick up my friend Laura and have, like, five joints pre-rolled, and we'd smoke them all. Always music mad loud: We'd go out to Long Island, get on the Belt Parkway, and go all around the edge of the city. At this point I would also do a lot of chair dancing: It was like a paraplegic dancing, only from the waist up, no leg movement. It was just all about face and shoulders, just winding your body. We were high, and we thought it was funny.

After the Caddy I had a green Chevy Lumina. This lady who lived in our neigborhood was selling it, and I grabbed it up because I'd broken the Caddy. I only had that for about a week before I crashed it. I hate cars with too much electronic shit: I prefer analog cars. I'd like a Barney Rubble car–you have to start it with your feet. I currently have two analog Beamers, but those aren't great smoking cars. They're too small: They get baked out really fast–windows up, you literally can't see out of the car. And you don't want to have the windows open. An ideal vehicle would be a jeep: There's tinted windows in the back, it's spacious, you never know what's going on in a jeep. To me a jeep is the same thing as an SUV–everything bigger than a car is a jeep. It's my mother, she does that: To her, everything bigger than a car is a jeep.

PRO TIP: To make your own smoking vent in the car, open one window so that the smoke gets vacuumed out. In my car it's the driver's side window, so I can monitor the situation. You have to be able to gauge the scenario, always looking in the rearview mirror at your friend with the blunt in the back, yeah, yeah, keep it low.

P.S. I don't want to get into a car where someone who is too stoned is driving. I don't trust anyone to drive stoned but me.

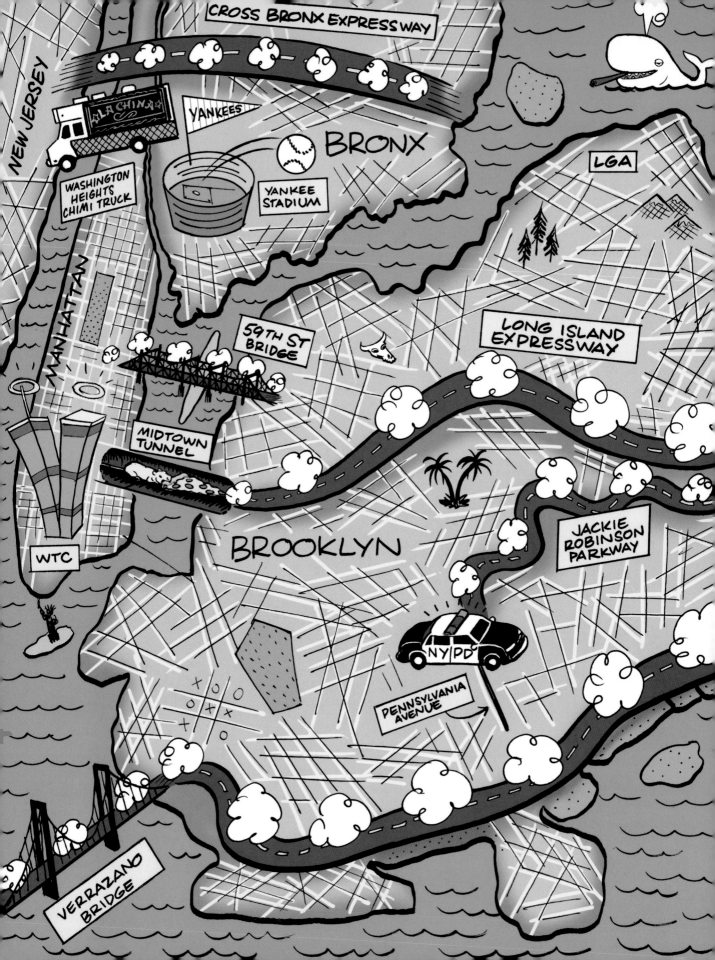

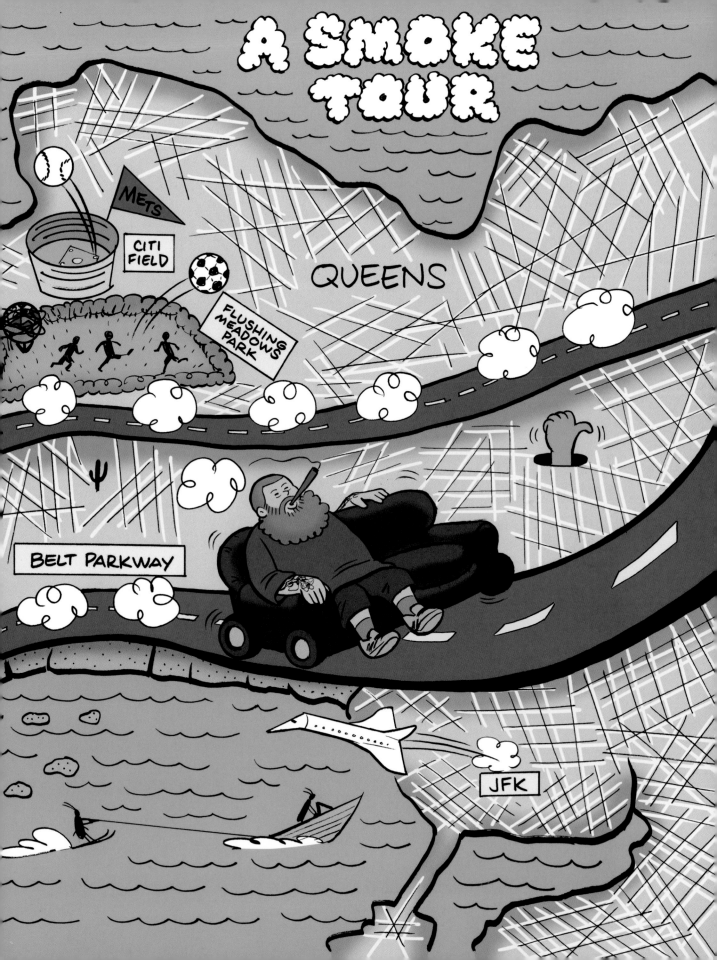

52. ICES

Ices are a huge thing when you're high. Whether it be the long ones in neon colors, the childhood legend from the bodega—it's amazing that twenty-five cents will buy you something so delicious. (It shocked me when I saw them not-frozen in the supermarket for the first time—it was like seeing my favorite ballplayer not in uniform.) Then there are the Marino's Italian Ices, in the little cardboard cup. The key to the Marino's, if you're a fucking purist, if you're a master connoisseur, is that you get it melted just enough so that you can flip it over inside the cup to reveal the crystallized gooey icy underneath part. Something happens down there; it's phenomenal. If you don't know about that? Usually what you do is very gently excavate around the melting edge to create the perfect icy bite, like you're an archeologist trying to find a new archeological site or trying to preserve the wing of a ten-thousand-year-old bird. Then you flip it. Sometimes I can't wait, and I literally go in when it's rock solid and I try to jostle it out with a very big spoon, or sometimes I get a knife and try to chisel it out. And, seriously, that shit should not be a rock—it's not venison that you hunted for and you're keeping it frozen for a year.

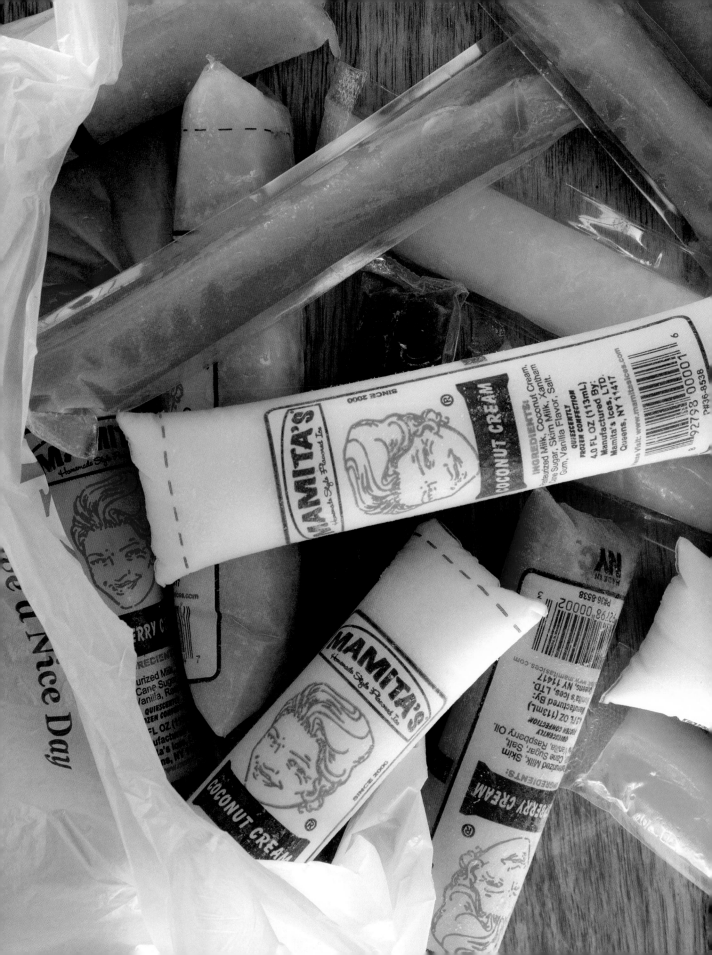

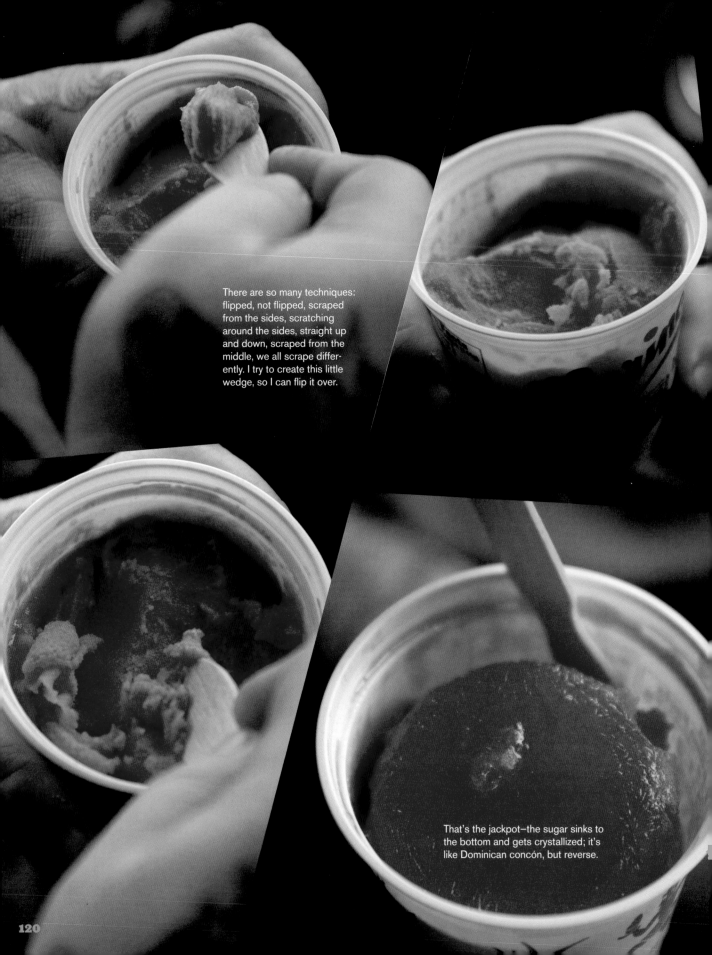

There are so many techniques: flipped, not flipped, scraped from the sides, scratching around the sides, straight up and down, scraped from the middle, we all scrape differently. I try to create this little wedge, so I can flip it over.

That's the jackpot—the sugar sinks to the bottom and gets crystallized; it's like Dominican concón, but reverse.

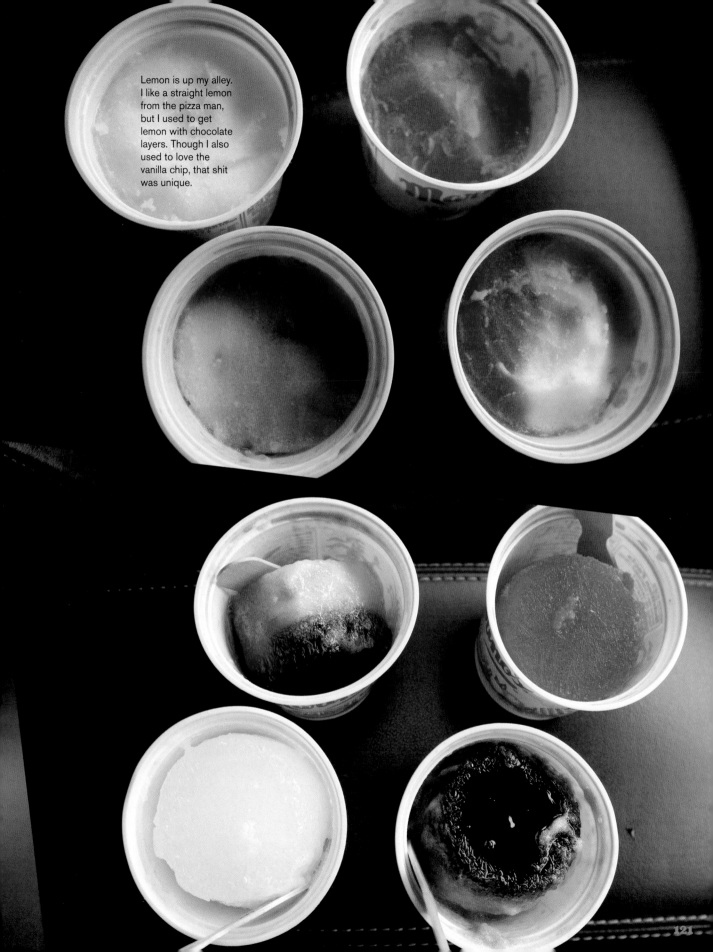

Lemon is up my alley. I like a straight lemon from the pizza man, but I used to get lemon with chocolate layers. Though I also used to love the vanilla chip, that shit was unique.

53. Spinach Pie

This is not quite spanakopita, and I can't really call this Albanian *pite*, or I'll get in trouble. This is a recipe I have been making and making and perfecting until it is really next level. I learned from watching my grandmother, but this is my own thing, and I've really got it down to where I want it: I promise you, this will be the best you ever had. The way my grandmother used to do it was to butter each layer of phyllo dough, brushing it and flicking it and painting the butter on in circles. I use olive oil—I use almost an entire bottle of olive oil, true, but that's OK; you want this to be amply tasty. I use beautiful baby spinach, and you don't cook it first. If you do that, it's no good, it's just going to be a pile of poo—in most spinach pies the spinach is the worst part, a tight little layer, but not this one. You could add parsley—my grandmother would—but I don't fuck with parsley like that.

Serves 6–8

1 pound (455 g) baby spinach
1 large white or yellow onion, diced
3 cups (720 ml) heavy cream
2 large eggs
½ pound (225 g) Bulgarian feta, crumbled
Flaky sea salt to taste
1 25-ounce (750-ml) bottle really good
  extra virgin olive oil
1 pound (455 g) box phyllo dough, defrosted
2 tablespoons sesame seeds, optional

1. Preheat the oven to 400°F (205°C).

2. Put the spinach in a very large mixing bowl and ever so gently crush the leaves with your hands, just a little bit. Pile the onions on top and add the cream, eggs, cheese, and a heavy pinch of salt.

3. Mix everything together with your hands, like you're dressing a salad—you want everything mixed together and every leaf to be coated in cream. Taste the creamy sauce—it should be nicely salty, so add more salt if needed.

4. Coat the bottom of a large lasagna pan with a lot of olive oil, about ¼ cup (60 ml).

5. Lay down 4 sheets of phyllo dough across the bottom of the pan, then drizzle oil over the top, using the back of a spoon to spread it around. (You don't have to oil them one at a time, because it'll soak through.) Lay down another 4 sheets of phyllo dough across the bottom of the pan, again covering them with oil, then repeat this process with 4 more sheets. (If the sheets break or tear, it's fine.)

6. Use your hands to mound the spinach mixture in small fluffy piles all across the bottom of the dish, doing your best to get all the pieces of onion and cheese and a little bit of the juice. Just don't throw away the creamy liquid left in the bottom of the bowl: Whatever sauce is left you pour over the top of the pie, so you get the edges sealed with the good, good taste. And why not add some more olive oil, if you want?

7. Top the spinach layer with 4 sheets of phyllo dough, again covering them with oil. Repeat this process twice more, so that you add 8 more sheets of phyllo dough to the top of the pan. (At this point, you can just go ahead and add any remaining phyllo sheets you have to the top of the pie if you like it extra crispy, or not.)

8. Tuck the phyllo dough in around the edges of the lasagna pan, and baste the top with lots of olive oil. Then pour the leftover spinach-cream liquid all around the edges of the pan—a few little pieces of onion or spinach in there are fine. Then let the corners drink up a little more olive oil, for good measure. Now tilt the pan slightly and swirl it around, so the oil and cream mix a little, covering the top. Sprinkle with sesame seeds, if desired.

9. Bake this for about 45 minutes, checking in at around 30 to see if it needs a little drink of olive oil, if it looks dry.

10. Remove from the oven and cut slices as you go. Eat this hot, at room temperature, or cold straight from the fridge.

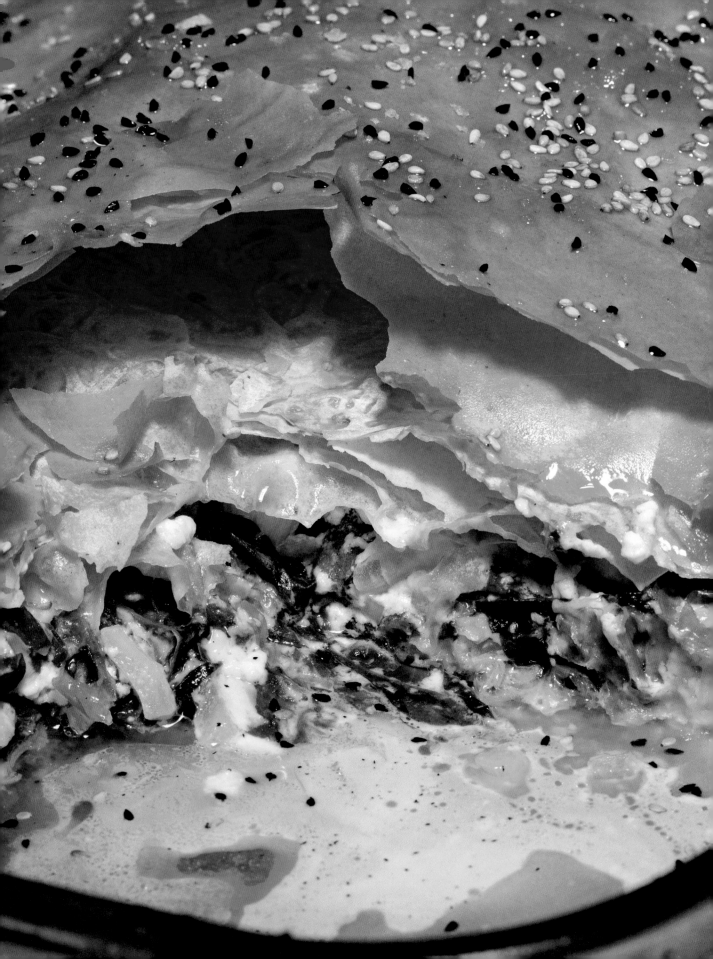

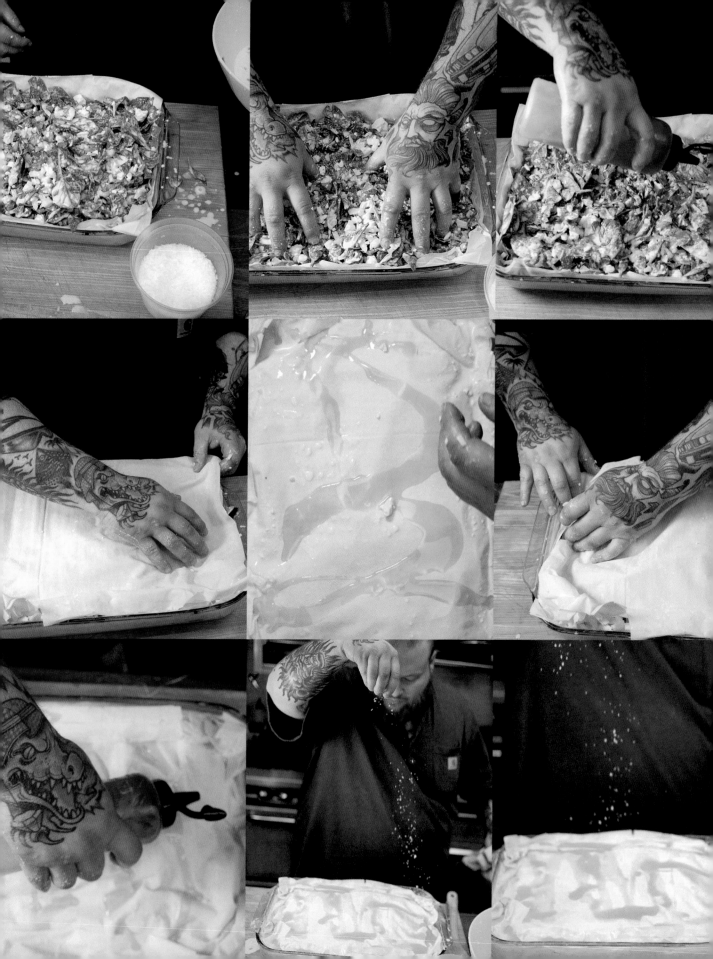

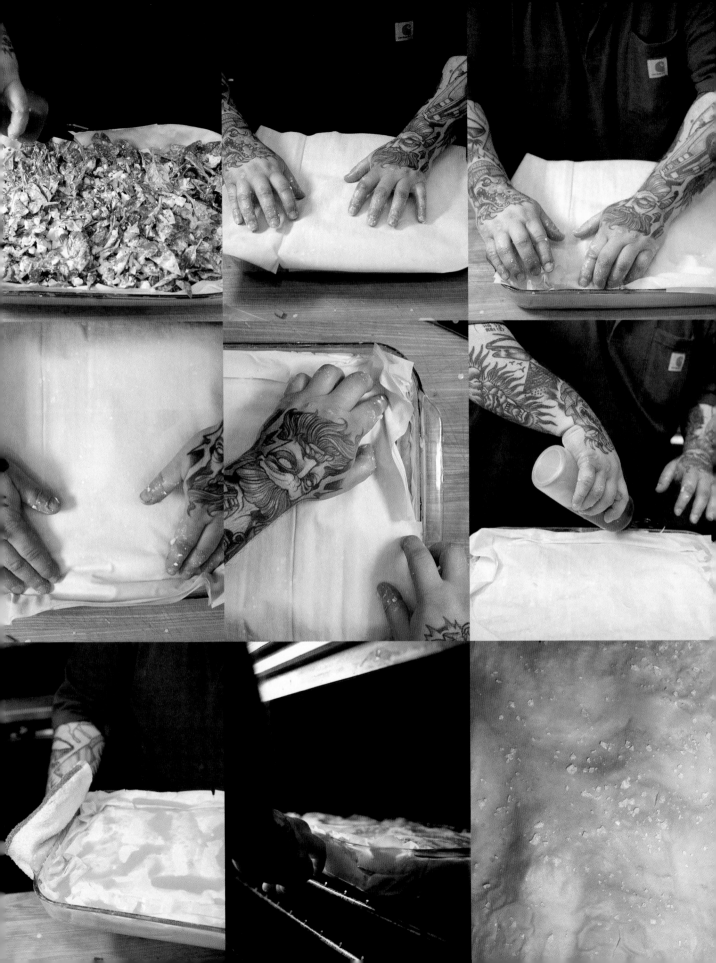

54.

Playback: 3:43 P.M., September 8, 2017, Action Takes a Hit

0:00 (silence)
0:01 (silence)
0:02 (silence)
0:03 (silence)
0:04 (silence)
0:05 (silence)
0:06 (silence)
0:07 (silence)
0:08 (silence)
0:09 (silence)
0:10 cough
0:11 cough
0:12 cough
0:13 cough
0:14 cough
0:15 cough
0:16 cough
0:17 cough
0:18 cough
0:19 cough
0:20 cough
0:21 cough
0:22 cough
0:23 cough
0:24 cough
0:25 cough
0:26 cough
0:27 cough
0:28 cough
0:29 cough
0:30 cough
0:31 cough
0:32 I've never had so much flavor
0:33 cough
0:34 cough
0:35 cough
0:36 cough
0:37 cough
0:38 cough
0:39 cough
0:40 cough
0:41 cough
0:42 cough
0:43 cough
0:44 cough
0:45 (takes another hit)
0:46 (sounds of inhaling, water moving through glass)
0:47 (sounds of inhaling, water moving through glass)
0:48 (sounds of inhaling, water moving through glass)
0:49 (sounds of inhaling, water moving through glass)
0:50 (sounds of inhaling, water moving through glass)
0:51 cough
0:52 cough
0:53 cough
0:54 cough
0:55 cough
0:56 (silence)
0:57 (silence)
0:58 (silence)

COUGHING TO GET OFF-ING

You have to cough to get off is what I've been told, by the old-timers. You're not really high until you cough, they say. I know once I cough, I start tearing up, it's hell, yeah, there I am. You've come to terms with where you are, or like that montage where you start floating in a sea of fucking stars and shit. It's a beautiful feeling.

0:59 (silence)	1:21 cough	1:43 (silence)
1:00 (silence)	1:22 cough	1:44 (silence)
1:01 (silence)	1:23 cough	1:45 (silence)
1:02 (silence)	1:24 That was an unbelievable flavor	1:46 That one made me cry
1:03 (silence)	1:25 (silence)	
1:04 (silence)	1:26 (silence)	
1:05 (silence)	1:27 (silence)	P.S. Have we talked about coughing
1:06 (silence)	1:28 (silence)	and pissing at the same time? It's
1:07 (silence)	1:29 (silence)	a crazy thing, if you're a dude. You
1:08 (silence)	1:30 (silence)	know you got your joint in your hand
1:09 cough	1:31 (silence)	and you take a hit while you piss,
1:10 cough	1:32 Wow	and you cough and it goes all over
1:11 cough	1:33 cough	the place, not to mention it hurts.
1:12 cough	1:34 cough	Coughing and pissing is no good.
1:13 cough	1:35 (silence)	It can get messy. It can damage the
1:14 cough	1:36 (silence)	urethra. (Also if you run the water
1:15 cough	1:37 (silence)	while you're pissing, it makes you
1:16 cough	1:38 (silence)	piss harder.)
1:17 cough	1:39 (silence)	
1:18 cough	1:40 (silence)	
1:19 cough	1:41 (silence)	
1:20 cough	1:42 (silence)	

55. Win Son's Milk Bun Ice Cream Sandwiches

This is one of my favorite stoner foods, from this Taiwanese place in Brooklyn called Win Son. The owners came over to my studio and made these for the Super Bowl. I had this same combination of soft bread and ice cream in Naples—it was brioche with gelato, gently warmed. The basic Win Son milk bun ice cream sandwich is made with a humongous slab of ice cream, buttered peanuts, and condensed milk, but we went crazy: slices of cheesecake and fruit jams from pages 30 and 32, the caramelized plantains called maduros, sprinkles, olive oil, crumbled cookies, whipped cream, mint. It's maybe not easy to make milk buns from scratch, but it is fun to put them together. And once you have that dough, you just freeze it, and then you have milk buns ready to go straight into the fryer. They can be used for a whole fucking slew of things: You can start stuffing things into them, making, like, barbecue buns or fried chicken buns. You can just buy a bag of buns from a Chinese bakery too, or good brioche—we give you an out, to be a sad stoner bastard on the couch.

HOW TO MAKE A WIN SON MILK BUN ICE CREAM SANDWICH

1. Get an Asian milk bread roll and split it in half, like a burger bun. You can find milk bread from all kinds of Asian bakeries in all kinds of shapes and sizes—and flavors, too, like green tea and sesame. You're looking for a roll shape, a bun shape, but two slices of a milk bread loaf would work too. The dudes from Win Son fry their dough instead of baking it, so you can too if you make your own,* but the non-fried baked kind is gonna work too. So would a round of brioche or a nice, soft, sweet, yeasted dinner roll.

    * Trigg Brown, the co-owner of Win Son, says home cooks should try the recipe from TheWoksofLife.com, just make them big enough for the ice cream and fry them instead of bake them.

2. Take a pint of your favorite ice cream. Make sure it is nice and frozen. Use a sharp knife to cut the bottom off the pint, cardboard and all, so that you're left with a 3-inch (7.5 cm)-tall circle at the top of the pint. Remove the cardboard from the circle and place it gently inside the milk bun. You can keep the bottoms to make the sundaes shown on pages 80 and 81 the next day. I did.

3. Top the milk bun with condensed milk and crushed toasted peanuts tossed in a little melted butter with a pinch of salt.

4. Repeat with more ice cream and buns, adding layers of your choosing, such as the whipped cream you make for my Banana Pudding on page 35, olive oil, sprinkles, cookies, the jams on page 32, the cheesecake on page 30, or maduros. You don't know how to make maduros? First, to make maduros, the plantains must be fully black, not yellow, not speckled, but black-black—like, moldy. You'd almost think they were too ripe. So if they're not black, step one is to wait until they are, that's the way. Now peel two or three plantains and slice them lengthwise into three long slices. Put a good amount of oil in a medium skillet, a nice thick coating. Vegetable oil—this is the one thing I don't want to make with olive oil; it just doesn't taste right. Now start cooking the plantains over medium-low to low heat. You just have to go slowly with these, or else they'll seize up and never get soft. They'll taste okay, but they'll never get soft. Then you just let them cook and cook till they're soft. Now it's like plantain custard, like some totally different thing. They are also amazing on their own with sea salt, a combination I tasted for the first time at a Nigerian family's house outside London.

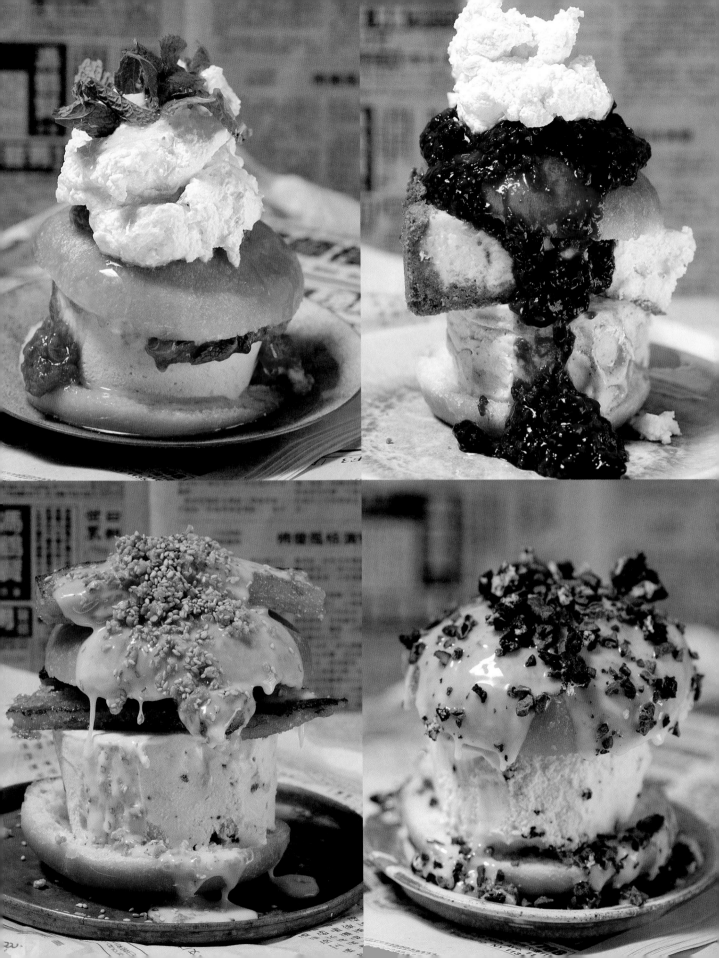

This was right before we got on the airplane and left LA, after doing extensive research for this book. This blunt contains four different flavors from Nameless Genetics, including a super super Mega Wellness that was like the thee-times OG; rotten cherry; and a sunset sherbet mega lime cross that was next level. Then I put down a entire flat sheet of rosin that we had and I just laid it on top of the weed paper, so the rosin was encapsulated in the blunt. That shit fucking lasted forever.

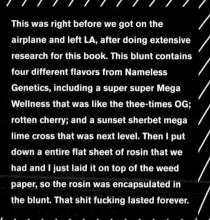

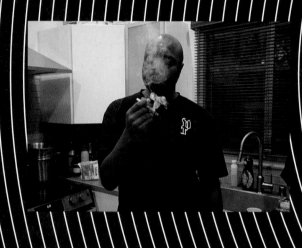

A Note on Seshing Dynamics: When I travel, I tend to curate hotel room or Airbnb seshes, where I have old friends from the cannabis community. Sometimes you create connections. Sometimes you can't have the same crew at the same time cause they're beefing. Even in the cannabis community, there's always some issue, and it's like high school shit, especially with social media. It's like when somebody got invited to sleep over and you didn't get invited and they tell you, *yeah, I was there* and you weren't, and it was so sad, you know, 'cause you really wanted to be at the sleepover.

56. Seshes

* From the Wiktionary: sesh
(plural seshes) Noun. 1. (colloquial) A period of
time spent engaged in some group activity.
2. (colloquial) An informal social get-together or
meeting to perform a group activity.

Sometimes at a sesh
there's mad weed left
over all over the table,
and I just take my arm
and sweep it off, just
throw it on the floor. I
remember how I used
to do the opposite, to
search and find the
weed on the floor.
It's disgusting. Not
searching for the
weed on the floor—
what's disgusting is
that I throw it there.

131

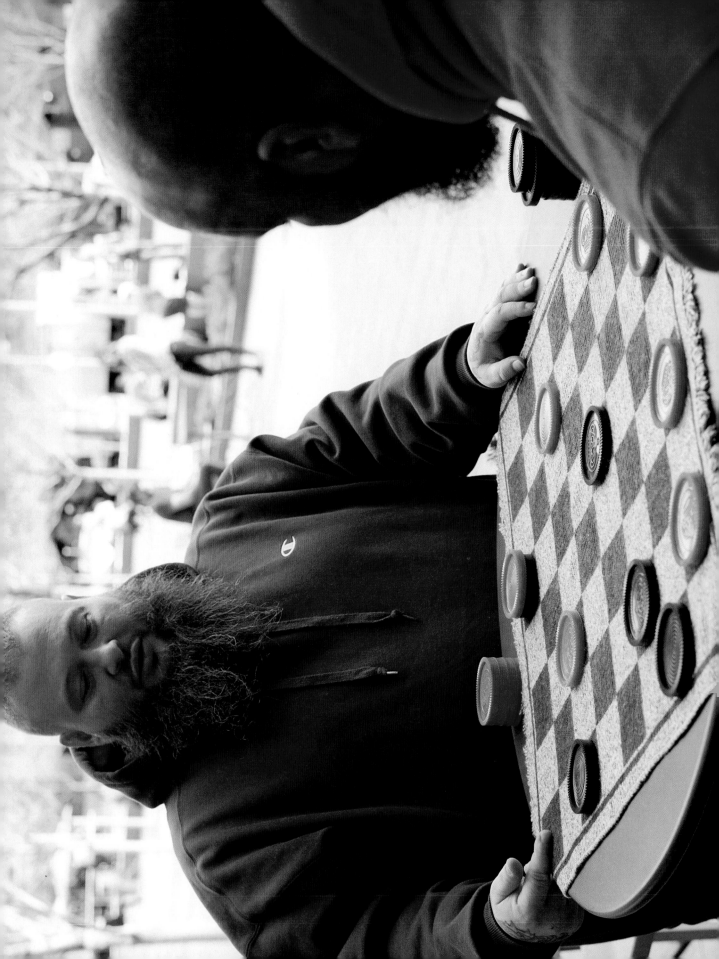

57.

You know how much fun it is to play sports while high? You have so much focus, it's so much iller, you feel like you're killing it. There's just something about being stoned and swinging the bat at a baseball or at a softball, or shooting hoops or playing handball or riding bikes, surfing, or any shit like that. And being stoned out of your mind while swimming? There's pretty much nothing like that, being in a body of water, when humans are mainly water. We are water, and then we're in some water? It's crazy, like pizza on top of pizza. With any kind of physical activity—even cleaning the house, which is amazing while high—the weed homes you in, and it gives you an edge, this "Eye of the Tiger" type of feeling that you don't have usually. When I smoke and I do things that are athletic, it makes me so much more focused, almost as if I am there with the ball going through the hoop when I shoot the basketball, with pinpoint accuracy. And then you get the victory blunt when you're done with the whole entire night. That first blunt right after you're done, when you light it up, it's like, **win.**

Sports and weed has always been a big part of my life. I used to play softball on Sunday mornings all summer long: I was a pitcher on the team, and I also batted either second or third. Each game consisted of getting nice with your boys beforehand by smoking a fat blunt. It created the camaraderie, and sports is all about camaraderie. A good team has chemistry, and that's why a good team always gets high together. True, sometimes I smoke during the game, but it was really that fat blunt before the game that would have me focused.

For a long time, handball was also the thing. Handball is a New York City game: There were several parks where people played, and we'd travel to P.S. 200, P.S. 164 to play, Austin Street at the park in Forest Hills, or the overlook in Kew Gardens. Smoking weed and handball is the perfect harmonious symphony. It's really the perfect game not just for getting high, but to listen to music to, to drink beer to. It's competitive, but you'll still see dudes say, **yo, let me get a hit of that cigarette.** Sometimes, they'll even start playing with the cigarette in their mouth.

With handball, I used to be really good: corners all over the place, hitting rollers. A roller is where it hits the bottom of the wall where it meets the floor and the ball just rolls. That's, like, the ultimate shot in handball, because you can't hit it back, there's no way to physically get it, it's like a home run, a grand slam. Whoever hits that shot is the winner of the shot. We used to play mad games of handball, get high. Then play more mad games of handball, get high, go get an iced tea. Play mad games of handball, get high, go get a slice of pizza. That was it. That was summertime.

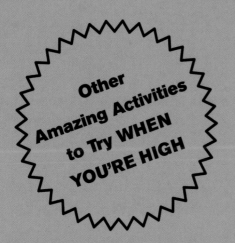

Other Amazing Activities to Try WHEN YOU'RE HIGH

58.
DO GRAFFITI, DRAW, SKETCH, PAINT, OR DOODLE

Graffiti and weed go hand in hand: It's like activity and art. I prefer to do graffiti in the daytime: Nobody thinks it's illegal if you're doing it in the daytime. It's like, eh, must be some artist. But if you're out at nighttime, it's illegal. I learned that from *The Art of Getting Over*. Doodling, drawing, painting on any surface, such as a pizza box, is also ill.

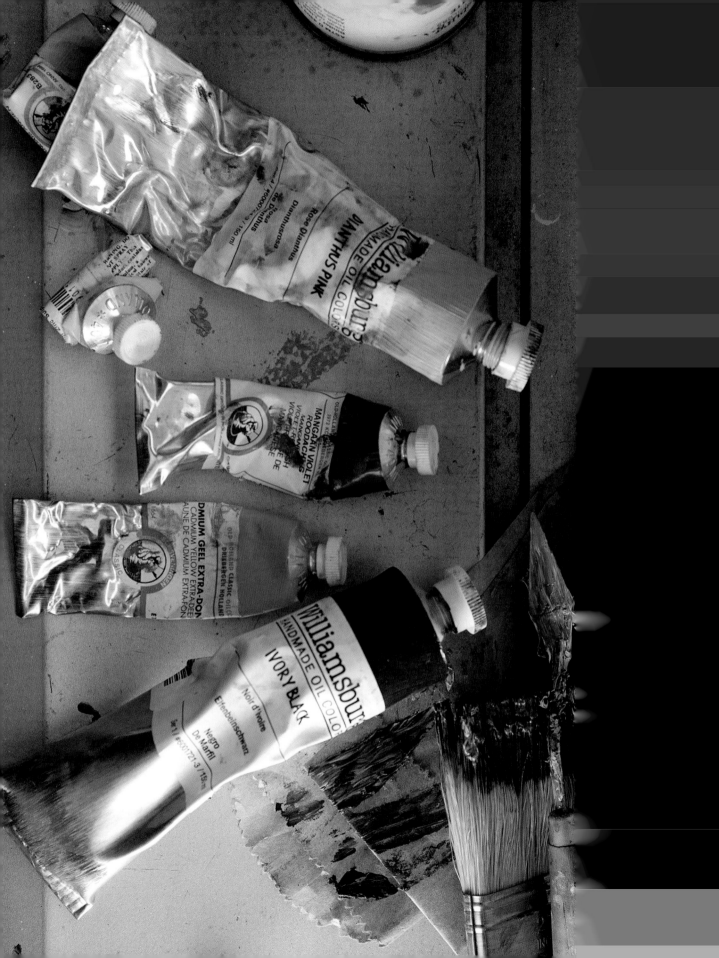

59.
THROW POTTERY

Like in *Ghost*. Throwing pottery is fucking sick. I like to leave it rustic, with the marks from your hands still in it. I was thinking about carving it like the way crystals are faceted. It's not only fun, it's really therapeutic. Do it by yourself with your headphones on, like running.

60.
MASTER IKEBANA, THE JAPANESE ART OF FLOWER ARRANGING

I learned from a woman in the Queens Center Mall. She told me I was a natural.

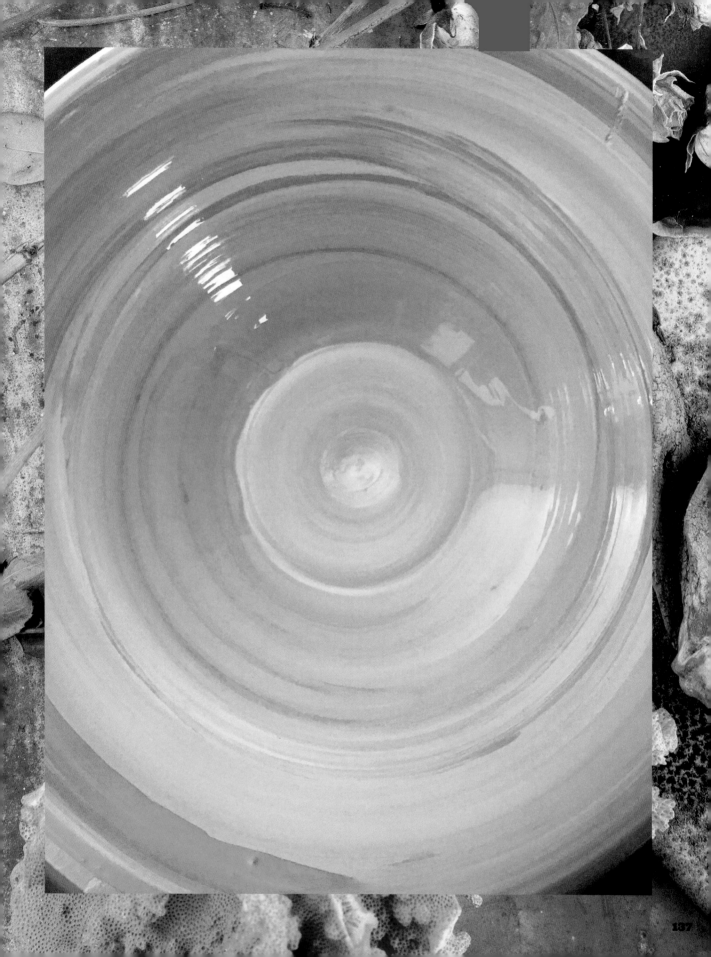

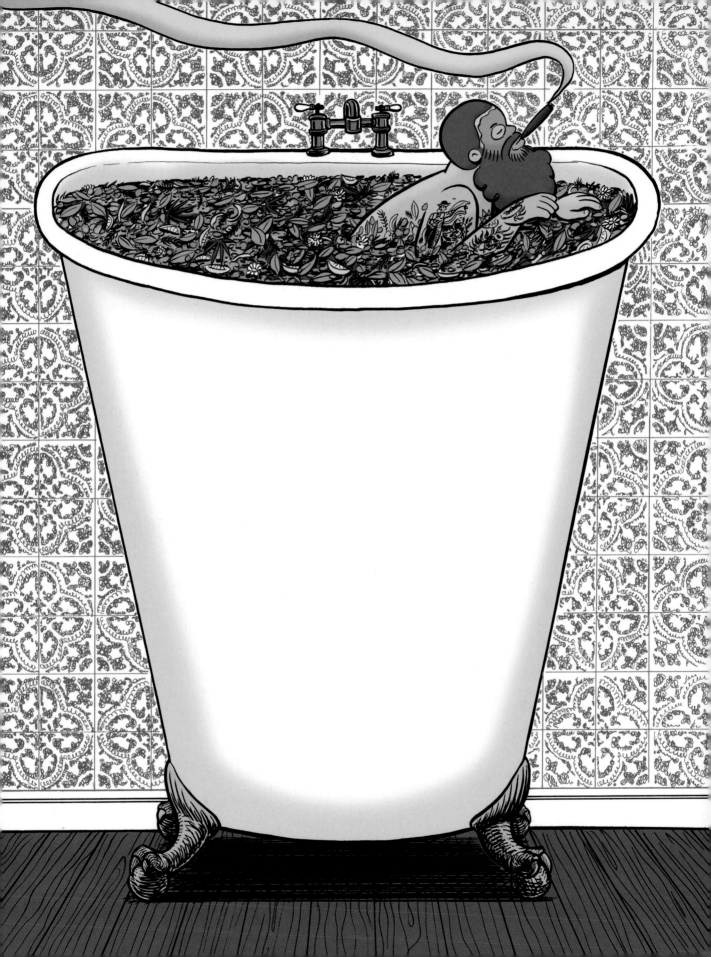

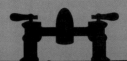

61.
Take a Seasoned Bath

I love taking seasoned baths, with tea and rose petals and orange peel and the green clay on my face looking nuts. Then I drain the bath and I turn on the shower, because when it hits me from a higher angle, it's like rain. I look like I'm in fruit salad. Showering in extremely hot water when you're stoned is also super heady. Let it run on the back of your neck between your head and your shoulders: It transports you to another place for some reason, perhaps the future. You go through a time portal, the time-space continuum, a wormhole, a portal to another galaxy. You know what's incredible? To get stoned out of your mind, really fucking good, really, really medieval stoned, and just fucking turn all the lights off and shut the door and take a bath. It's life-changing silence. It's fucking next-level sensory deprivation.

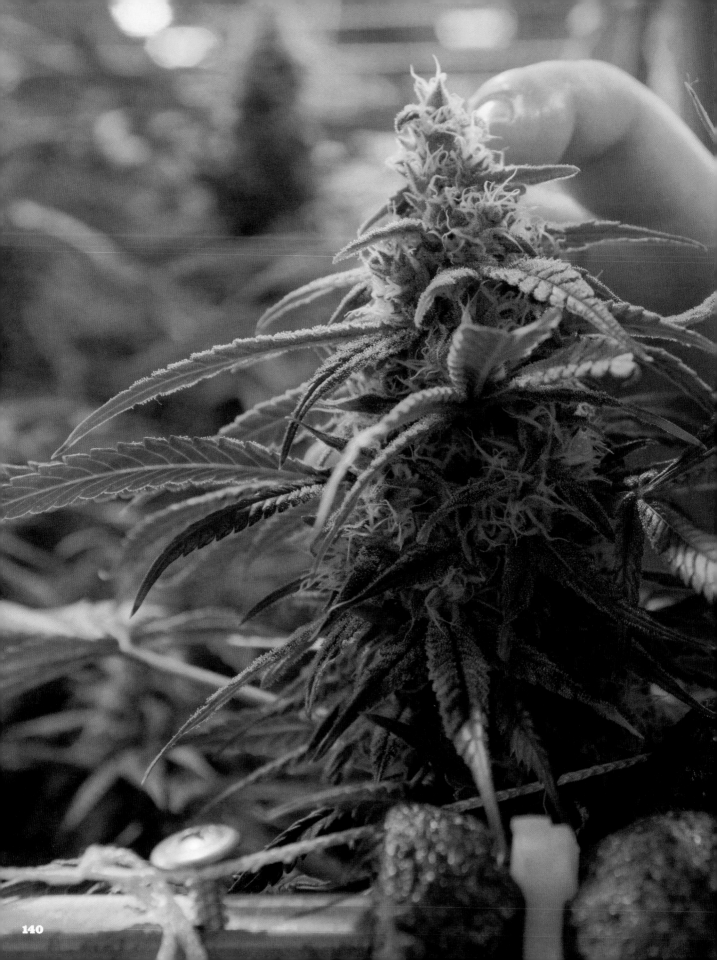

62.
GOOD WEED

My thoughts on good weed are somewhat dated, partially because I didn't grow up on the West Coast, having everything at my fingertips. I grew up having to buy it off the street, not even knowing the name of it. The way that technology has gone, the advances in botany and the way growing and processing the plant has evolved, it seems that we obtained the knowledge to make this plant more powerful and more giving within the past fifteen or twenty years. I don't know if that's the case, but it seems that way to me, in my world. You can also share knowledge now; it's more open, not taboo. There's knowledge out there for everybody through their computer.

When I started smoking what I thought was good weed, the B.C. or Beasters from British Columbia, it was just the first "dro"– as in hydro weed, grown hydroponically. Now that I have become a connoisseur and gathered more knowledge about that shit, I know it is disgusting. Now there's always a new flavor, a new strain; every minute a new kind of flower is being born. When I was growing up, there were only a couple of types of weed, just a few different flavors. And if I am really being honest, really early on there were no flavors; there was just weed in a bag.

Then came the Beasters, tight, rock-hard nugs of green shit with yellow hairs all over it: It looks nice, but these days it sucks in comparison to everything else out there. That's what was around for a while, until we got the "exotics," the "exos." That meant you didn't really know what it was: The question wasn't what it was or where it was from or who made it, like it is now, but could you even get good weed. Back then I was lucky to have the connect, to know the dude who had the connection. I started smoking good weed then–good for the East Coast in the late '90s and early 2000s–and haven't let up since.

We used to go to Ridgewood, and they had, like, ten different flavors of weed in these jars. And then there was this company called Cartoon Network in Long Island; you would call the number to the Cartoon Network and meet them wherever to go buy weed, and they would have a bunch of different shit. That was, like, crazy, you know, like holy shit, what are we doing right now? We're driving my friend's white Pontiac Grand Prix with some shit written on the side in grafWiti font and then smoking dumb weed from the Cartoon Network. Because our goal in life was to smoke as much weed as possible.

Later there was hash–the first time I had hash was 2001–and then there was kief, which is when you just run good weed through a screen to take all the THC crystals off the weed. The first time one of my friends had a big jar of kief, we thought that was some specialty shit.

Since then I've transformed so many different times. I used to put oil and extracts in joints first: I was making joints like crazy, I was just putting so many things in there. This hash, that hash. Make it look like a fucking tie-dye blunt. Then I had to make snakes out of hash, so it looks like the line where the shit is in the shrimp. One of the methods of using old-world hash is you make it into a little thin snake, then you lay it into your joint. In 2013, when I was at Al's house in LA recording Rare Chandeliers, I used to make, like, four or five joints with this new style weed, new style hash, and lay them in, so it kind of looked like a gun barrel.

Now new weed is some next-level shit. I just learned about most of it myself: They have reinvented weed; weed has been updated in a phenomenal way. I am now the most stuck-up weed connoisseur: I want to get new weed from reputable botanists and people who are straight up about clean medical stuff, everything grown unbelievably clean and organic, no bullshit added, and smoke it out of a gorgeous glass pipe. It's, like, so far from where I was when I started, it's crazy.

Beginning of Time

| Jamaica Avenue brown weed | Beasters & Exos | Pude/Haze | California*, Kush, Cookies, Earwax, etc. |

700 billion years ago, in the times of dinosaurs

Post-Pangea, pre–modern civilization

World War Two

Westward Expansion

*Somewhere around this time I was one of the first to have their own vape pen, a.k.a. the G Pen.

The Finest One Billion Percent Organic Most Flavorful Terpiest Hash That I Press into Rosin & About 10,000 Other Strains of Beautifully Grown Weed

The Renaissance

End of Days

My New Weed Glossary

BHO: A type of extract made with butane oil. Pushing butane through glass pipes and freezing out all the terps. *Shatter, budder,* and *wax* are usually referring to BHO. Traditionally BHO gave you more yield and more terps, but the trade-off is, you're using chemicals. I only buy BHO from one guy, who has the process down to a science; he vacuums it all out, all of it.

Cannabinoids: These are chemical compounds in weed. People like getting stoned, people like getting high, but weed's also got medicinal purposes; they found that it helps so many different conditions, you know. You usually hear about THC, as in tetrahydrocannabinol, which is the one that gets you high, and CBD, as in *cannabidiol,* which works as a relaxer, as an anti-inflammatory and anti-anxiety aid and so on. But THC can also be a healer. But once you get into it, there are lots of others, like THC-A and CBD that do different things when combined in different proportions.

Cannabis community: There is a community of people who love this shit and support one another—people who appreciate glass, people who appreciate botany in general, people who appreciate healing, shit like that. From all walks of life. There's supporting the community and being a part of the community. I am part of the community. There are also cannabis community celebrities, like glassblowers and hash makers and kids who take dabs on Instagram, and wooks all over the world.*

* See the "Wook" Look Book, page 164.

Dab: You're just putting a literal dab of any kind of a pure weed extract in a glass pipe or dry heater and smoking it, a.k.a. taking a dab.

Extracts: This is modern hash. The first time I heard of an extract, it was called earwax, and it was some little greeny-yellow shit that I used to just sprinkle into the joint. Extracts are modern concentrates of the good stuff, the resin—the oils and chemical compounds— that come from the trichomes. The crystal-y, sticky things you see on plants—that's it; that's what gets you high. Weed is good, yes, weed is greeeat, but there's no way that's better in modern times in my opinion than to smoke really clean extract. You know how you only need a little touch of vanilla extract? It's the same thing, it's so potent and powerful. (But sometimes you want the vanilla bean, there's no doubt about it.)

The roots of extracts are in the original kief and hash, both of which are just the sticky chemical compounds collected from the plant in some manner. Kief you get just by collecting what fell off or by sifting weed through a screen, which is why some people used to say they were smoking screen. And hash is kind of just a lot of that, all pressed together. You used to smoke hash on a hot knife, which is like the original dabbing: Heat the knife, the hash would smoke, you inhale it, get high. Every herb has some oils, like the way mangoes and limes are sticky right off the tree, or plants that are fuzzy, you know. They exude. If you keep that plant pristine, you can collect that oil, extract it. I've

heard that in the mountains where weed was originally grown, there's a lot of old-school ways of making hash: just running your hands along the plants, and whatever was stuck to your hands, that was the hash. That's like natural extracts. I haven't seen it done, but I can imagine just running your hands over a field of sticky bud like that.

Today they get those oils from the plants in many more technologically advanced, more precise ways, and they call the results extracts. That's why I feel anything that's not weed is just hash, in some form. If it's not weed, I call it hash. Extracts can be called various things depending on their texture or how they are made, like rosin, live rosin, sift, which is like powder, ice hash, ice oil, wax, oil, shatter, budder, diamonds, which are big hunks, sauce, which is saucy, sugar, where it's buttery but crystal-y—these are all different stages of extracts. The whole thing, it's very similar to candy making: It's all about temperature and how you bring it to where it's at. To get it to that shatter form, you have to put it to a certain temperature, then you have to whip it into butter. Then you have to do something else to get it to something else.

Everyone has their own techniques for making these; everyone has their favorite to consume. I used to like budder a lot, when I smoked BHO, because I love terps, but solvent-free gets terpier all the time as people get better at making it. (They used to say budder has the most terps; it "locks them in.") There are even

people who don't care about flavor; they smoke distillate, or pure concentrate of THC, where they take garbage weed and they make it into a flavorless THC oil. So it's mad potent, but it has no flavor. You just take a hit of that and you're fucking washed. New shit gets invented every day. Now they got these things called space rocks, which are disgusting, where you take weed, you dip the entire weed bud in oil, and then you cover that in kief, so it looks like a powdered doughnut.

Glass: A glass water pipe designed for smoking extracts. (There is also a dry heater, which is a glass pipe that doesn't use water.) It's called a rig or glass or pipe or a piece, not a bong. It's an oil rig: It's basically a water pipe designed for smoking oil and extracts. It's a piece of art, really, and it's better than art. Can you smoke a Picasso? I don't know the exact origin of the modern glass pipe. From what I heard, they came from Vancouver, from BC Bubbleman, who makes mesh screens for making extracts. They say his sister was a glassblower who made him a pipe. But Bob Snodgrass was the Eugene, Oregon, godfather glassblower who started it all in the 1970s and taught nearly everyone else how to do it, including Washington state glassblowers like Scott Deppe, who cofounded Mothership Glass, which created technology that revolutionized the game (like the Klein, a circular way of recycling water in a bong), and taught the next generation of blowers, like Kevin McCulley, a.k.a. Quave.

Glob: A glob is a huge-ass dab. Like something that's ridiculous. Unnecessary. I glob out. I do. A glob is a normal size for me. But I take normal pinches also: little pieces, a little touch, a nib.

Regs: Terrible weed. I used to be able to get an ounce of regs for fifty bucks. It stands for Regular, but you could also call it Trash. Or Garbage. Bullshit. Harrachs. Boo Boo. Doo Doo. Anything that you could make up that sounded terrible, that's what you could call terrible weed. I don't know where Harrachs came from. They do have some decent regs: your greens, your browns. Brick weed. Jamaican weed, Mexican weed. You know, some of the Jamaican shit is good; it's called Tyson, 'cause it knocks you out.

Solvent-less, solvent-free: This is the real modern boutique artisan hash, as in not using any butane or other chemicals. In a way, everything has reverted to the old-world style of original hash making. This is usually made with just ice and water, so the crystals and oil stay intact and can be screened out of the plant matter. This is all-natural shit. You tend to get a little bit less, and you used to get less THC, but that's changing as people get better at the process. People want clean stuff; they don't want bullshit. The more knowledge everyone has, the more this type is going to grow, as it's more natural and healthy. Bubble hash, water hash, and ice hash are all types of non-solvent hash—then you usually press it through a filter one more

time again to get the purest stuff, which is the cleanest way to dab.

There are all kinds of machines and spinners and shit to help in this process now too, but at the end of the day I don't even want somebody spinning my shit. I want somebody doing it by hand, and I want to meet them. Just like with food: You want a machine churning the butter, or you want an old woman you've seen doing it by hand? What sounds a million times better? You want the old woman. I am all about this kind of boutique, artisan weed—that's all I smoke, and that shit is expensive. I'm the type of a guy who becomes submerged in a type of thing. If I like a wine, I want to meet the winemaker, look at his grapes (ha ha), look at his vines, get to know his family. It's the same thing with weed. And the best way to ensure that you have the finest stuff, that you're not inhaling any garbage, is if you know who grew it, who processed it with only water and ice in an organic and fucking healthy manner and then delivered it fresh frozen to you, because it has to be frozen or it gums up and becomes one ball like hash, so it's sent freezer-packed, just like Omaha steaks. And it'll last mad long frozen as long as it's in the freezer or fridge, and then you just press it out as you need it.

Strain: A strain is a flavor of weed. Some strains are the original as found in nature, but most are crosses created by growers. People are inventing new strains all the time. And there are strain hunters, dudes who travel to Afghanistan or Morocco or wherever

and come back with smuggled seeds so that they can grow them or bring them to a grower. There're people who have plants for years and years and years that they use to grow, or they make babies called clones to grow from or give to other people.

Good growers are like winemakers these days; they take care of their strains, protect them, grow them with specific temperatures and soil and water, and they get crazy with the names of their strains. It's no longer just Sour Kush or Haze.* One strain I have is called Cherry Pie Dogshit. It's a cross of a strain called cherry pie and another called dogshit—it smells like dog shit, but when you hit it, it's like you're eating a blue Tootsie Pop. *Bro, that smells like fucking dog shit*—boom, that'll be the name of the strain. The new marketing scheme these days is to name weed after food: Cherry Pie. Cookies. Gelato. Sherbet. Orange Creme. Birthday Cake. Lemon Peel. Garlic Mushroom Onions, or GMO. It's usually because these weeds have similar smells to whatever is in those foods. That GMO, it really is like fucking mushroom gravy coming out of your nose. I love it. I know people who can't even speak in normal human talk, only strain names and terps. It's like music people who can only talk in references to Bruce Springsteen in 1988.

I have one strain right now that I think is the best strain I've ever smoked that I just call Rosewater. I was in Portland when I tried it the first time. It's a mixture of three things: Cindy 99, Skunk, and some other shit. That shit makes me want to fucking cough. It's dank: sweet and moldy but gorgeous like my favorite kind of wine, which is from the Zibibbo grape and pink and bubbly and sweet and tart. But really, there is no one best strain. Anything can make me happy at any moment. You taste something fucking amazing, and it's like the wind just hits you: *Ahhh . . .*

      * **Haze:** Haze is from Washington Heights, which is why we sometimes call it the Uptown. We don't know where it comes from originally, but we've never had that flavor anywhere else. Originally they would never sell it to me. They thought I was a cop the first couple of times because I speak Spanish. If you go up to Washington Heights and you speak Spanish, they think you're a cop. Body usually goes and gets it, 'cause he knows them. Then Body would come back with fifty dimes. The first place we ever found out about Washington Heights was from this dude named Genie, a graffiti writer who was a big pothead and always had weed. He put us on to Uptown. After that it was a wrap: When I was around eighteen I would go uptown with my boy Con, literally we'd make two or three trips or day, or even four or five, 'cause we'd get it for other people. People would give us their money, and they'd sell it to Con, and I'd ride up there with him. Somehow we'd get extra weed for ourselves, so we'd find people with cars to take us back and forth with other people's money. That was pretty much the MO every day for many summers: Smoke weed, drive back

and forth up to Washington Heights to get Haze, paint graffiti all day long, chill, and play handball, every day. That drive was the best: Take the LIE, take that shit all the way over, take it for free over the Fifty-Ninth Street Bridge, get the FDR at Sixtieth Street, go right uptown. Then we'd hit the Dominican chimi truck directly after getting the Haze. It was so close that someone would be rolling the blunt while the chimi was being bought, as we like to multitask. Everyone has a job: I would roll the blunt.

Terp: A terp is really a terpene. There are lots of *penes*, but this is the important one. Terpenes are found inside things like weed, fruits, flowers, or the hops that you use to make beer. They are aromatic chemical compounds that you smell even more than you taste, found in the oil glands in the trichomes. The better weed is grown, the more terps it has and the better yield of cannabinoids it will have when you squeeze it out into oil or hash. A lot of terps also means lots of flavor. Some people say terps may also have their own therapeutic benefits. With weed, a terp is kind of like a flavor profile, like tangerine or mushroom. (I always question people who don't like the smell of weed. It's like not liking the taste of cilantro. I get it, but it's weird to me: The smell of weed just tastes so good.)

    I first started hearing about terps in the last three years; before people started extracting things I had no idea what they were. It came around with the age of extracts. Now it's slang, as in,

I am all about the terps, which just means that you want that fire flavor, or even that you are super stoned on good weed: You're terped out. When somebody makes good oil, it's, *oh, he got the good terps*. Actual heady bro sentences: *I am so used to the loud terps, I can't fuck with the rosin.*

Trichomes: These look like little crystal-like hairs, usually purple or orange, coming out of the plant. Those are where most of those good chemical compounds and oils and terpenes are coming from. Sometimes trichomes look so intense close up, they look like those skinny Asian mushrooms. Good weed has lots of these—the plant produces more oil and trichomes when it's colder, so indoor growers know exactly how to lower the temperature to produce more. In the olden days this type of shit wasn't as developed as it is now: I don't even know if people were looking for that to happen.

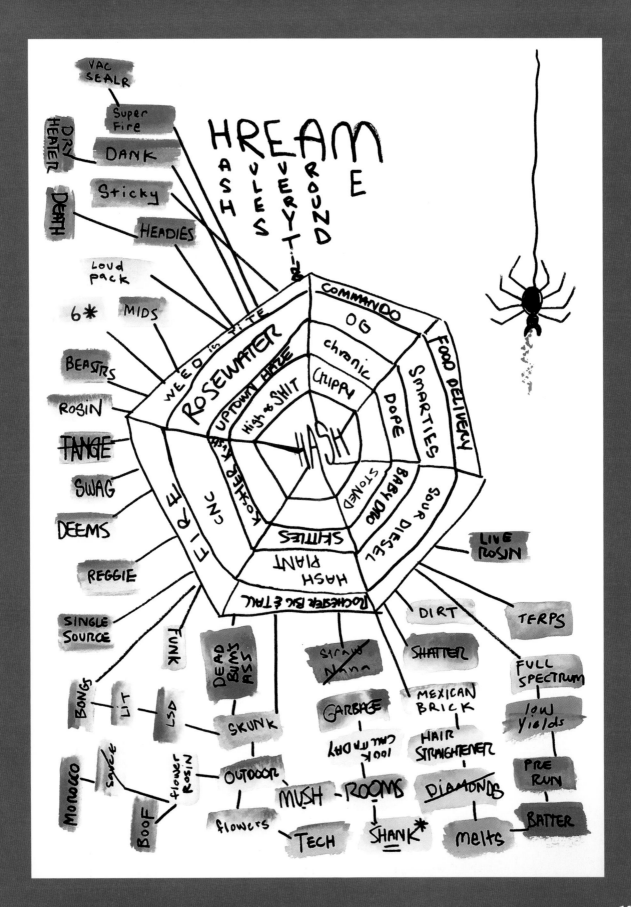

147

Whenever I go on tour or travel anywhere, the minute I land, the good weed should be waiting. I don't care about anything else except that there is good weed waiting. If we stay in a shitty hotel room but there is good weed, I am much more able to deal with it than I would be if it was a shitty hotel room without good weed. Luckily my friends and I are savvy: When we want something, we usually are able to get it. With our combined efforts and outreach and Instagram, hitting various people up in various ways, we usually figure it out, and in each new city we find the weed shaman, the one with the access to the really good weed and the local cannabis community.

Sometimes it takes a few days: The South Africa trip I took a few years back was bleak until we found our shaman. He was a guy on a motorcycle, wearing a fucking earring and a tank top. We were all on mushrooms, and when we went into his house, we started cracking up, because he had a giant folding fan on the wall, as if it was art, and **The Simpsons** figurines in a fish tank. He was a friend-of-a-friend-who-knew-somebody, and we met him after all our other leads had slipped away. We'd already had some kids go try to buy some bullshit weed just to meet us. I appreciated their effort, but they brought **le garbage.** I mean, it was trash, worse than brick weed,* I mean the worst weed ever–I think I got a fever smoking that weed. But then our shaman came and shamanized us out; he showed us the light. That's one of the other things the shaman does: shows you the light and opens your mind to make you happy.

Shamans do amazing things. In Rome I have a shaman with three fingers on one hand; he calls himself the Claw. In Norrköping, Sweden, I have a shaman who hid weed in a little drainpipe in front of the hotel for us. And sometimes the shaman finds you. In Australia, I was fiending out of my face for two days, just walking out on the street in pain, and, what do you know, a fucking dude just pulled over in a Maxima and was like, **Yo, Bronson, holy shit, I can't believe I see you, dog. Yo, my boy's been wanting to give you some oil.** I had seen nothing but bad weed, so my shaman presented me with good weed and a pipe and oil for dabbing. And they brought it to me and we seshed.

Not too long ago I landed in Miami after a thirteen-hour trek from France, and we met a shaman–he could be considered a savior, as they are one and the same–at Mary's Coin Laundry, which is also a Cuban sandwich spot, with a little window where you get takeout and one table with an umbrella. He had a chicken sandwich with croquettes waiting for me, but the superstar that he is, he had the rig set up for me right at the umbrella table. I blasted off at Mary's right in front, then had that sandwich, and all the anxiety and angst from traveling went away.

Everyplace I go now, every venue I play, there's somebody waiting to show some sort of love with weed to shamanize me. Many people will wait backstage just to smoke with me once I am done. I've met some of the greatest people this way. Let me just give you an example: I was at Camp Bisco in Scranton, Pennsylvania. I've been to a lot of hippie shit, but that was one of the most hippie shits ever—you know, everyone is on LSD, everyone is dressed in tie-dye, kids have on fucking patchwork-woven pants. I meet this one guy who lives in Brooklyn, he's a nice guy, he was with this girl who was really into weed oil, she just wanted me to try her oils that were made in Maine. They were really nice people, so I have them backstage in my trailer, and we're smoking and dabbing and chilling. This is what these people wanted to do, just come join me and smoke, like-minded shit. So I do the show, I come back, and literally there we are in the same spot an hour later, smoking and dabbing and chilling. And then another one of his friends shows up who had a little LSD ruler tattooed on his thigh that shows you the perfect size for a hit, and then some other friends of his who came through blew glass, and they gave me a little glass pipe and a pendant.

* Brick weed: shitty weed with seeds from Mexico, pressed into a brick. Really good weed doesn't have seeds; that's why they call it *sinsemilla*: "without seeds."

Marc, my road manager, on finding the local shaman:

"With the dabbers, the heady guys, sometimes I've never even met them. I meet 'em on social media; we chat online, on different underground applications that I will not name. We communicate. In Europe specifically I have some guys I hit up, and they know everyone else throughout Europe, throughout the world, so they send the job out: **Yo, this dude's in town.** And some of these people haven't even met the guy I know, they just know about him from a mutual friend of theirs. So it's like three different me going through even know the people who don't guy. It's a wild community, and it's all a risk too, because we've never met these people. Some-times they barely speak English. Pretty much all of them are good: It's like a network. The guys that I meet, the reason you know that they're part of the community is be-cause when they come through, they either have a Pelican case with a bunch of stickers, or you can tell by their clothing. The hat. The pins. A pendant. Most of them usually have a pendant on. I'll know immediately who a person is just by looking at them. I was just in San Francisco, and we had to get butane, and I didn't know the location. And I saw this guy on the corner, and I was like, **Hey, man, I'm sorry, this is a random question, but any chance you know where to find butane?** He was like, **Hell, yeah, bro. Right down the block right on Haight Street there's a smoke shop.**"

63. Finding the Shaman   63. Finding the Shaman
63. Finding the Shaman   63. Finding the Shaman
149
63.

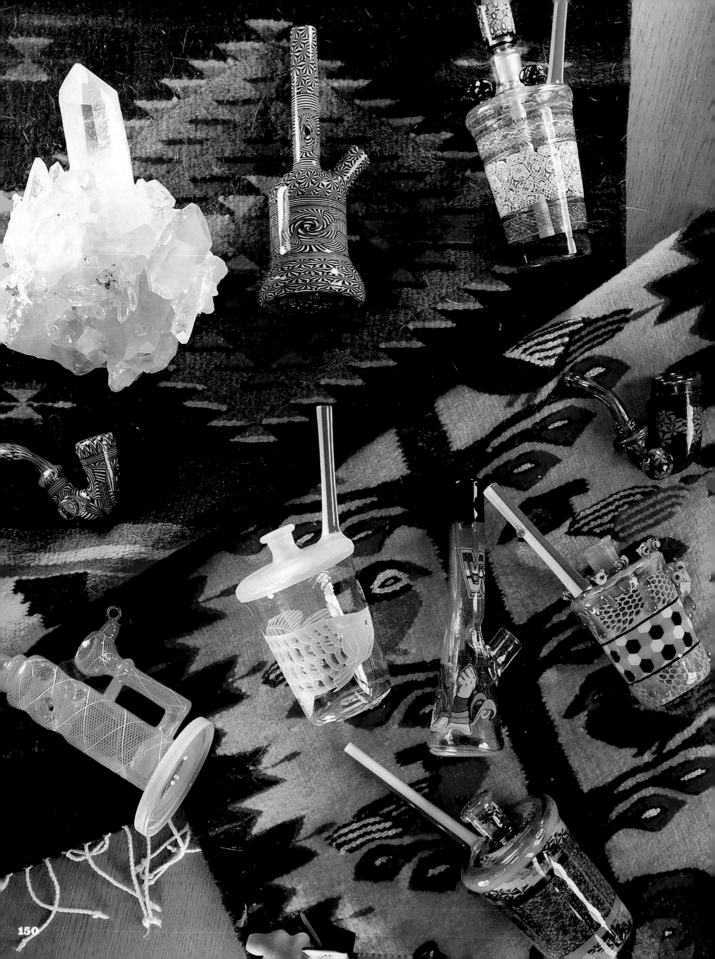

64.
The Importance of Bad Weed

Smoking all this good fucking weed these days has almost made me forget about the struggle: all the bad weed I've smoked. If you drew a map of everywhere I've had bad weed, it would be the world. Sometimes you have to smoke bad weed just to bring yourself back to reality, where you were. Just like anything, you have to keep yourself grounded, so you don't get too self-indulgent.

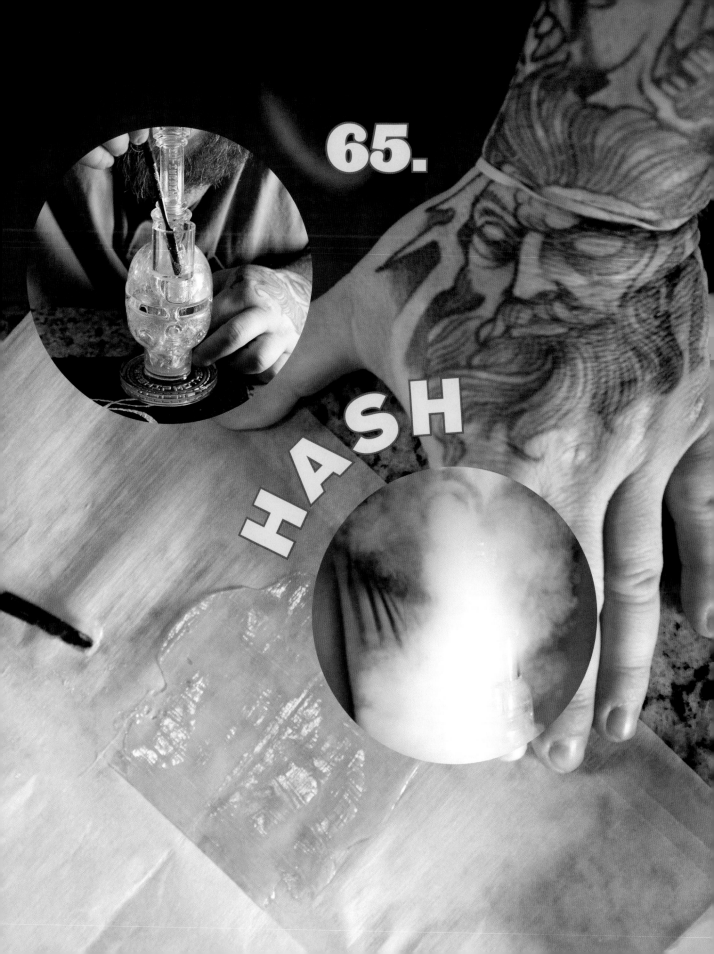

65.

HASH

Dabbing *modern hash—a.k.a. extracts, as explained in My New Weed Glossary on page 144*—is my preferred method of smoking weed right now. To me, it's weed in the purest form, the cleanest and most flavorful, and I usually know who grew the weed and how they grew it and what methods the extract maker used to make it. I love dabbing people out for the first time, when they have no clue what it is. A lot of my friends don't dab: When there's someone who dabs, I just want them to come hang out. Just please come hang out and dab with me. Nobody local dabs, so I either import them or export myself. Usually everyone else smokes joints or blunts, but I can't do that very often anymore. The added tobacco hurts my throat, and why mask the taste of the weed? It's burning the weed at a higher temperature, it's harsher, and it's less flavorful.

I also love the mechanics of using the glass pipe, pressing the dab, cleaning the glass. It's really a long process, but it's become a thing. It's therapeutic to me—I'm literally meditating every time I heat it up with the torch, put the timer on, getting the dab ready to go, hitting it at the perfect time, getting the flavor stuck behind my teeth. That's the way I gauge weed: If the flavor stays behind the teeth, it's stuck there, that's the fire. It's the whole process, starting with pressing the dabs from hash myself: You go through many steps and stages to get to the actual best product, the finest product that you could possibly get, and then it's just gone within a second.

The first time I ever dabbed was about seven years ago at a show in Utah set up by my friends DJ Juggy and Taskrok. Task is very educated about new trends within the cannabis community, and on that trip he said, *I got this shit, my boy's going to bring it through later.* In comes this dude in some baggy jeans, just a normal white guy from Salt Lake City. He has a glass pipe, the first dabbing rig I'd ever seen, a nail made of titanium with some crazy dome that went over it, a butane torch, and some yellow baby shit wrapped in parchment paper.

I'm like, *what the fuck is this?* I'd never even heard the word *dab* before.

But I was game: They gave me my first dab about an hour before I had to go on. You used the torch to heat up that titanium nail so hot, as hot as possible, *then you add a dab to the hot nail* and put the dome over the nail to keep all the smoke in. I take a hit, I inhale, and I'm instantly out of my mind, I didn't know what to do.

Now that was the old way of dabbing; we don't do it that way anymore. It took me a long time to get to the point where I am now, with dozens of rigs and nails made of quartz and a system and a refined technique: I didn't even know you were supposed to add water to the pipe at first, until someone was like, *bro, what are you doing?*

These days, you would never smoke it out of metal, or so hot. You let it cool down to just the right temperature, where you coax the flavor and the compounds from the hash. But that metal nail was the very beginning: It was like having the first Scion or Saturn.

I took a hit off that hot nail, and I coughed for an hour and a half straight, and that's not even an exaggeration. I was out of my mind, I couldn't take it, I didn't know where I was—I was fucked up. I had to perform, but there was no way I could perform. I got up there onstage and couldn't even get my breath. Two songs in, I was like, *yo, this guy fucked me up, he gave me the shit,* and everyone laughed. I stumbled off the stage, had a Coke at the bar, and the show was over. I've been dabbing ever since.

Note: My Wi-Fi password is *heady glass.*

HOW TO PRESS A DAB

BHO extracts are refined and can be fully dabbed, but for many solvent-less concentrates, such as sift or bubble hash, you'll really want to press them out through a coffee filter before you dab them to make them even purer and for maximum dabbability. You're essentially filtering them one more time. As I've mastered the press, I've kept adding to my process—I love the process. Now I want to press my dabs out as I need them; I want it fresh.

STEP 1.

Put a little of your concentrate in folded parchment paper and warm it up with a hair straightener, just until it becomes melty.

STEP 2.

Trim an organic coffee filter to a slightly rectangular square.

STEP 3.

Take the extract and turn it into a little slug, a little Tootsie Roll. Give it a fold into the filter, and roll it away like a little package, just big enough to fit right on the plate of a hair straightener. But remember it's very, very soft, so you have to be gentle. This is a fat one: I'm squeezing out a fat package.

STEP 4.

Cut a piece of unwaxed parchment paper neatly into a large rectangle.

STEP 5.

Place the little package in the middle of parchment, and make folds on each side so you don't lose any of your nectar—you're creating a nectar collector.

STEP 6.

This Revlon hair straightener is the one that I have to use because it's temperature controlled. It has a setting at 230°F, but it's not a real 230, it's like a light 230—it's kind of like 220, 210. You want to line up the nectar package on the plate and just gently press down onto the paper. Now if I go too quickly, it'll squish everything out, and that would ruin everything, you'd have wasted a lot of money, a lot of time and effort. So you get it started by hand, then you apply the woodworking clamp and start squeezing gently.

STEP 7.

Now it's just going to start oozing out, all that good poo poo. I like to move the clamp up and down to make sure I get full compression—you don't want to leave any nectar in the package. Open up the clamp and check, you look at your package, see if you missed anything, then attack the area exactly where you want to press. I am

pressing out some Wookies times Cookie Do. Cookie Do is Girl Scout Cookies crossed with Do-Si-Do, and Wookies is Cookies crossed with who the fuck knows.

STEP 8.

All my nectar is out of the filter and into the parchment, so I go over to the sink and drop the used coffee filter package into the sink.

STEP 9.

Now I make it pretty, make it nice, trim off the edges, flatten it out, and maybe cool it down to set it up by rubbing it with something cool, like chilled crystal, as sometimes when it's hot or humid it doesn't set up properly.

STEP 10.

Scrape off the loose little bits for yourself to dab and also to make it look cute, like a beautiful square.

STEP 11.

Trim down the paper accordingly, but don't trim too much at first because you'll be left with a weird-looking piece.

STEP 12.

Then it goes right into the freezer: It must be kept cold until you dab it.

> **PRO TIP:** You can press a dab out of an extract or good flower, but no flower dabs unless it is absolutely necessary, such as maybe one early morning in Rome when you have to call your dealer named the Claw to come over with some weed to a high-priced penthouse where a very famous random musician is playing show tunes on a grand piano. I saw my friend G.Z. do it first.

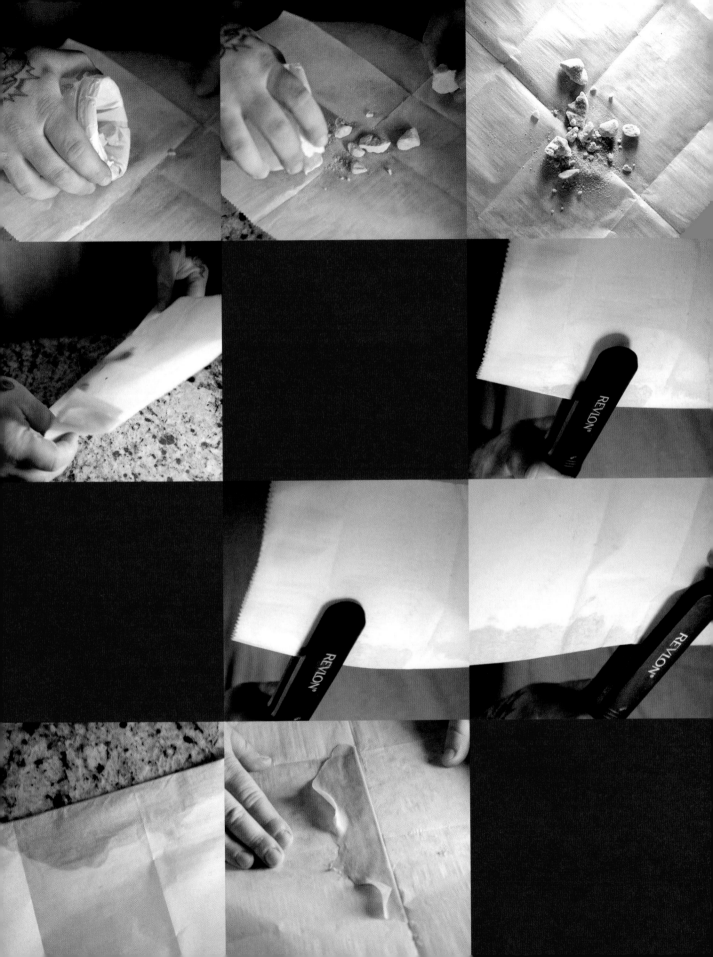

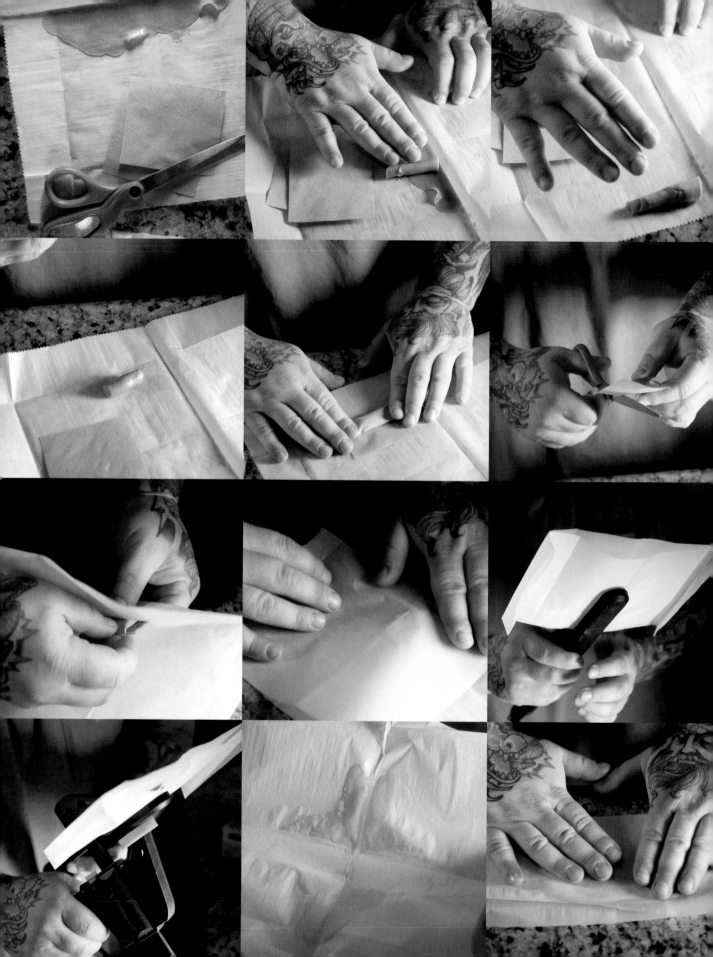

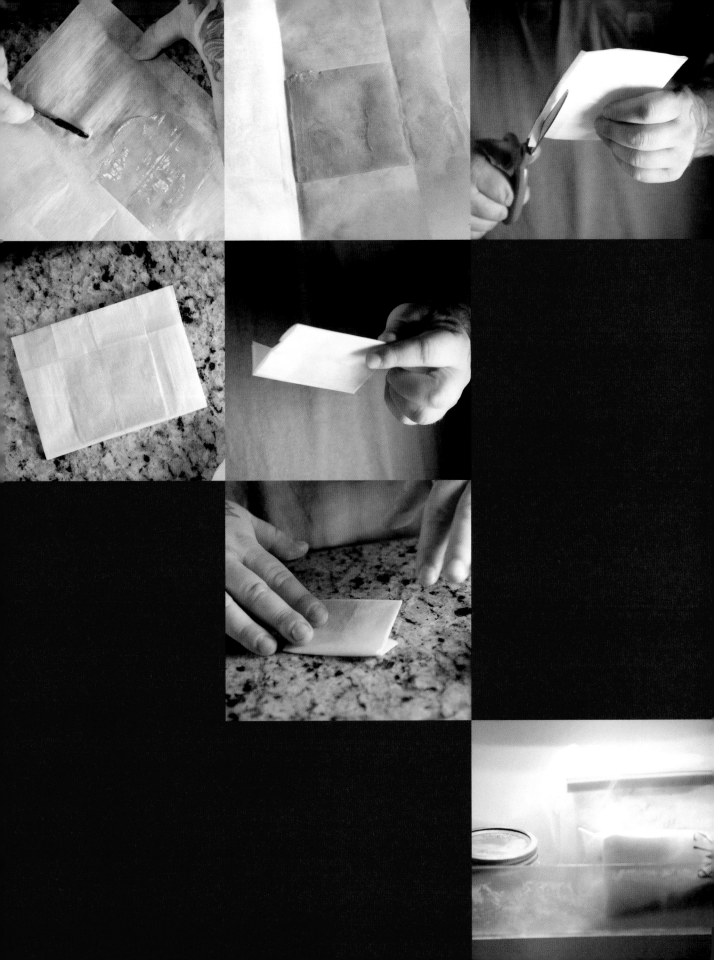

HOW TO TAKE A DAB IN FOUR PHOTOS

The pipe shown here is the Mothership Fabergé Egg, designed by Quave and Scott Deppe, with the *AB* engraved into it. This is one of my first pipes and a good everyday driver. I like to use a lot of different pieces all the time—I like variety, like I like my food, my beverage—but I hit this piece every single day. This was originally a floor model, being used by the guys on the job at Mothership. It was just a shop bong; this was the one they used because it had the best function. It is like driving a Cadillac: There're no flimsy little parts hanging off it, but it's a knock-around piece. It gives just this beautiful, breathy pull, nice and airy, with a little bit of resistance. It's just a pleasure, a fucking pleasure to hit this piece.

GEAR, AS SHOWN IN PHOTOS ON PAGES 155–159

- PARCHMENT PAPER
- UNBLEACHED COFFEE FILTERS
- SCISSORS
- REVLON HAIR STRAIGHTENER
- WOODWORKING CLAMP
- RIG (GLASS PIPE OF YOUR CHOICE)
- NAIL (AKA BANGER, PREFERABLY QUARTZ)
- CARB CAP
- DABBING TOOL
- BUTANE BLAZER BIG SHOT GT 8000 BUTANE TORCH
- BOUNTY PAPER TOWELS
- Q-TIPS COTTON SWABS
- 91% ISOPROPYL ALCOHOL

PRO TIP: HOW TO CLEAN A RIG

Water and weed stain glass, and it sucks to stain up a $50,000 piece of art. Plus when it's clean, it's art; when it's dirty, it's paraphernalia in the eyes of the authorities. So I have a technique, a cleaning regimen: I start by rinsing it with 99 percent alcohol first, and I make sure it's a little warm. Then I rinse out the piece with distilled water: It has nothing left behind, no residue, no trace of any mineral that can stain glass. Then I hit it with Palmolive Oxy. There's this little pump that sucks water in and out of a fish tank, a little mini-sucker, a little sucking pump to get the water out. You can put that in each of the openings of the rig, and it sucks all the water out and leaves you with a pristine dry pipe ready to be legally transported. I don't have that, so I place it gently someplace to dry. I used to just hang it upside down very carefully on my kitchen cabinet to dry it out, but then no one would be allowed in the kitchen, because it's a $50,000 piece.

I like to make sure every little nook and cranny is taken care of with my glass, and I like my dabbing tools to be surgical, just like a surgeon would have all his sterilized. It's a process, it's like cooking, it's like anything: Take the right steps, and the end product is going to be amazing. It's worth having clean glass; it makes you feel better, and you get higher. And I always do it myself: I took a rig to Venice once, and when it was time to go, I asked somebody to clean it out for me because we have to run, and I hear the water running mad hard in the bathroom. But I think to myself, *What's going on? The sink is not that powerful.* So I look in the bathroom, and there he is, cleaning the pipe in the bidet. *I said, Yo, throw that shit out the window, somebody's ass was on there.*

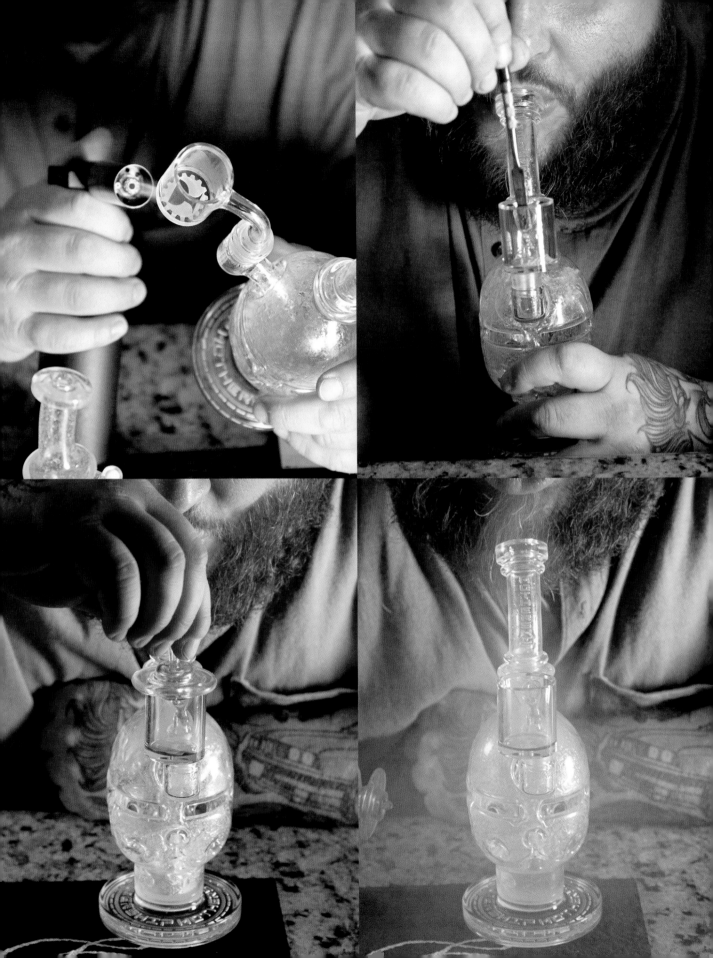

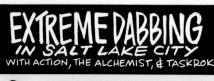

EXTREME DABBING
IN SALT LAKE CITY
WITH ACTION, THE ALCHEMIST, & TASKROK

WE GOT PICKED UP AT THE AIRPORT— YOUR BOY TASK. WE'RE GOING UP THE SIDE OF A MOUNTAIN—

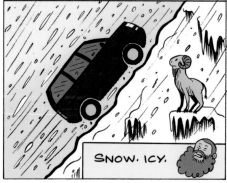

SNOW. ICY.

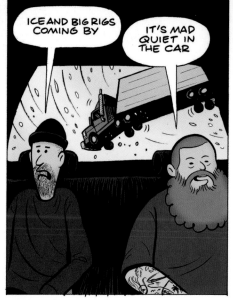

ICE AND BIG RIGS COMING BY

IT'S MAD QUIET IN THE CAR

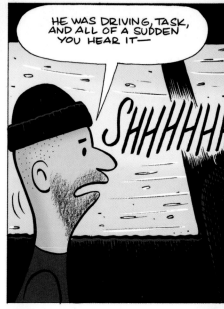

HE WAS DRIVING, TASK, AND ALL OF A SUDDEN YOU HEAR IT—

SHHHHHH

HE WAS TORCHING UP WHILE HE WAS DRIVING US ON THE EDGE OF A CLIFF!

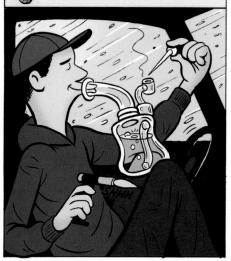

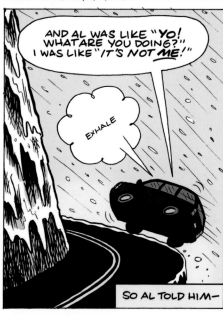

AND AL WAS LIKE "YO! WHAT ARE YOU DOING?" I WAS LIKE "IT'S NOT ME!"

EXHALE

SO AL TOLD HIM—

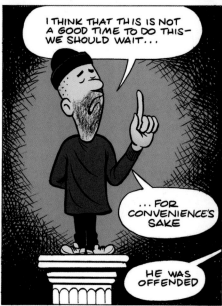

I THINK THAT THIS IS NOT A GOOD TIME TO DO THIS— WE SHOULD WAIT...

...FOR CONVENIENCE'S SAKE

HE WAS OFFENDED

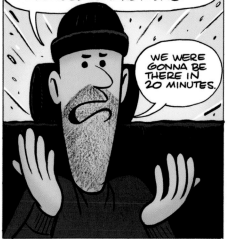

HE WAS! LIKE IT WAS TOTALLY SAFE— LIKE IT WAS A NORMAL THING! WHY— AT THAT MOMENT WHEN WE'RE GOING UP THIS ICY FUCKING MOUNTAIN— HE DECIDED TO TAKE A DAB.

WE WERE GONNA BE THERE IN 20 MINUTES.

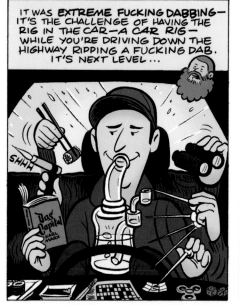

IT WAS EXTREME FUCKING DABBING— IT'S THE CHALLENGE OF HAVING THE RIG IN THE CAR—A CAR RIG— WHILE YOU'RE DRIVING DOWN THE HIGHWAY RIPPING A FUCKING DAB. IT'S NEXT LEVEL...

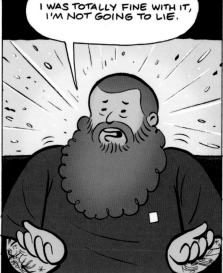

I WAS TOTALLY FINE WITH IT, I'M NOT GOING TO LIE.

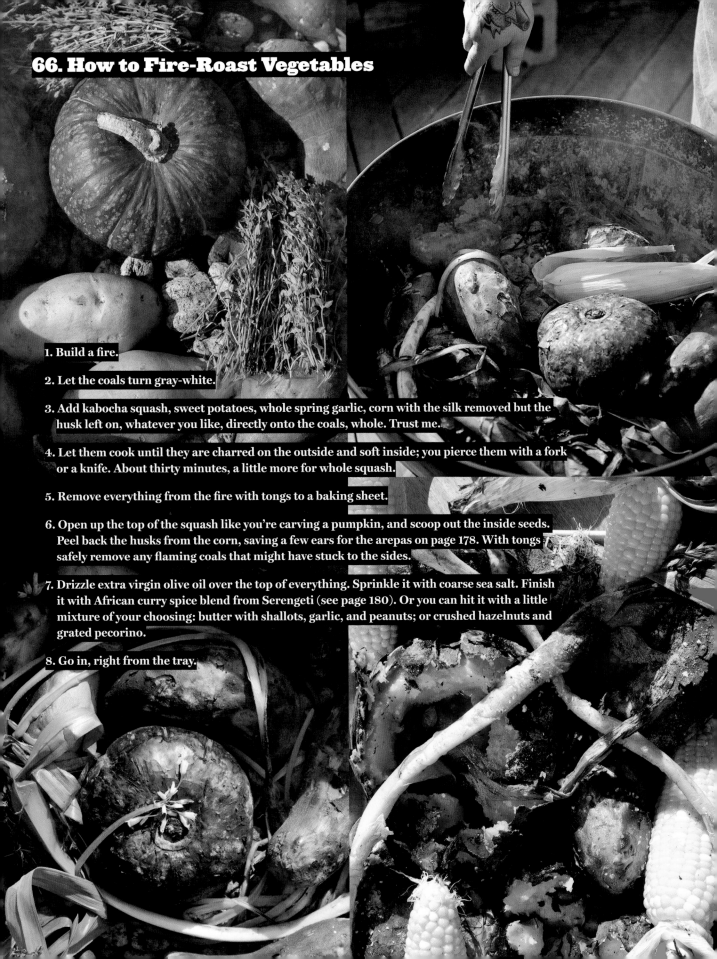

66. How to Fire-Roast Vegetables

1. Build a fire.

2. Let the coals turn gray-white.

3. Add kabocha squash, sweet potatoes, whole spring garlic, corn with the silk removed but the husk left on, whatever you like, directly onto the coals, whole. Trust me.

4. Let them cook until they are charred on the outside and soft inside; you pierce them with a fork or a knife. About thirty minutes, a little more for whole squash.

5. Remove everything from the fire with tongs to a baking sheet.

6. Open up the top of the squash like you're carving a pumpkin, and scoop out the inside seeds. Peel back the husks from the corn, saving a few ears for the arepas on page 178. With tongs safely remove any flaming coals that might have stuck to the sides.

7. Drizzle extra virgin olive oil over the top of everything. Sprinkle it with coarse sea salt. Finish it with African curry spice blend from Serengeti (see page 180). Or you can hit it with a little mixture of your choosing: butter with shallots, garlic, and peanuts; or crushed hazelnuts and grated pecorino.

8. Go in, right from the tray.

Muslim Lamb Chop

This was originally inspired by the Muslim Lamb Chop at Fu Run in Flushing, Queens, which gets braised and fried and smothered in a pile of Northern Chinese spices like cumin and Szechuan peppercorn and star anise, but I don't like star anise. It's also a massive chop, a crazy thing. This one is a baby, and it's fire-flamed, then hit with a bunch of spices I like from La Boîte (see page 210), especially dried Turkish Urfa pepper, which is black and sticky and smoky-smelling. Heady as fuck.

Serves 4–6

1 tablespoon whole pink peppercorns
1 tablespoon Szechuan peppercorns
1 tablespoon black sea salt
2 tablespoons sesame seeds
2 racks baby lamb chops, separated into individual chops (about 2½ pounds/1.2 kg)
Olive oil
2 to 3 teaspoons dried Urfa pepper
Flaky sea salt to taste

1. Light a fire in a barbecue grill and let it go until the coals are gray-white and hot. You want the grate to be right there on top of the fire, so that you can get a good char on your chops.

2. While you wait for the fire, muddle and crush together the peppercorns, the black sea salt, and the sesame seeds. It's meant to be a rough crush: You're just breaking down the peppers a bit, not making a paste. Set this aside.

3. Rub the lamb chops on all sides with olive oil, and sprinkle both sides lightly with the Urfa pepper and a little flaky sea salt.

4. Cook the chops over high heat, flipping them occasionally, about 7 or 8 minutes for medium-rare.

5. Transfer them to a baking sheet or some other kind of serving platter, and immediately dust them with the pepper mix, making sure to get both sides. These are also good with the pickled purple onions on page 178.

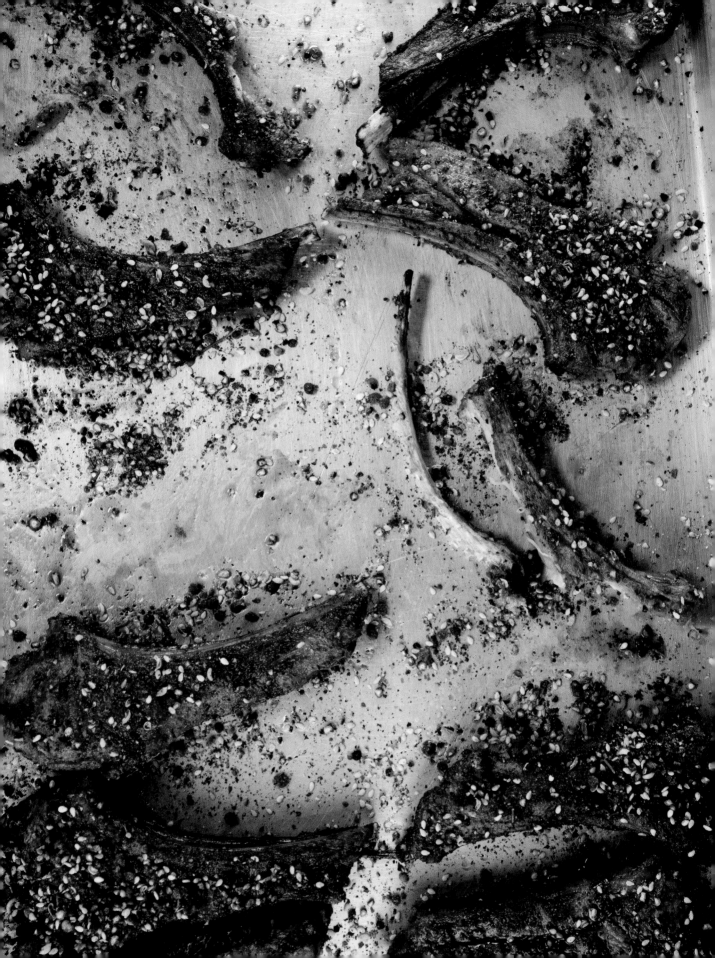

67. The "Wook"
Look Book

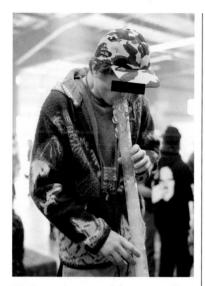

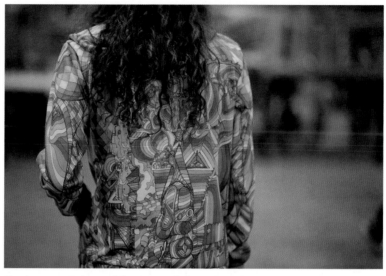

Nimin totatiam quam dolentem rero il ilignihil eaque volorionsed quam aut.

Sitatio eosant. Quias cus dolupti sum ut latiam commodicto volorerfero omnimin totatiam quam dolentem rero il ilignihil eaque volorionsed quam aut.

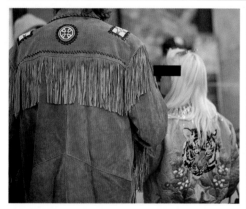

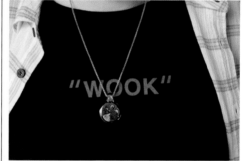

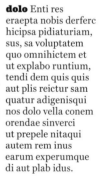

Nos dolo vella conem faceptas ut rem volentiatium autenis et qui il eost, ende laborest.

que Volora quamet modi ipsum hicabore volupti busaecus repel eum quature dolum ium vention sequibus et omnimpor as re, nonsecuptas neceatis natiae magnatis doluptat es ea si delignia.

dolo Enti res eraepta nobis derferc hicipsa pidiaturiam, sus, sa voluptatem quo omnihictem et ut explabo runtium, tendi dem quis quis aut plis reictur sam quatur adigenisqui nos dolo vella conem orendae sinverci ut prepele nitaqui autem rem inus earum experumque di aut plab idus.

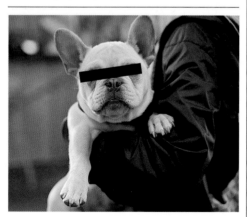

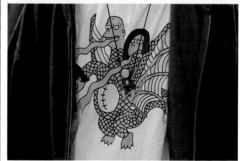

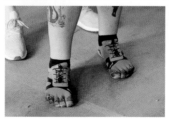

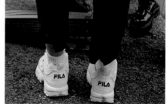

Dolum ium vention sequibus et omnimpor as re, nonsecuptas neceatis nat es ea.

Lo ma audit accae doloratem quam, omnis dolum, ut ut est lab id quam.

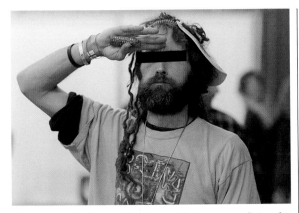

Sitatio eosant. Quias cus dolupti sum ut latiam commodicto volorerfeuam dolentem rero il ilignihil eaque volorionsed quam aut.

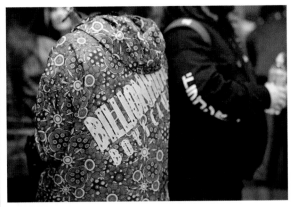

Vellicium idiam doluptam quodicitas dissundant fugiatur simaxim usandia coremolut. Eum quature dolum.

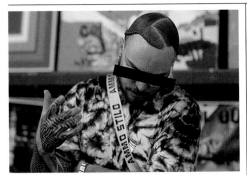

Coremolut mo comniendit plicipi caboreh enihicienet harchil molorest exeris ium.

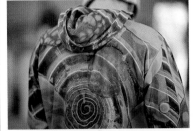

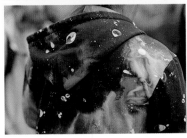

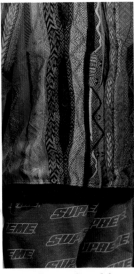

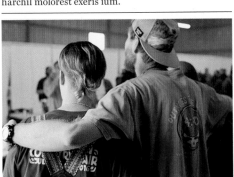

Restium isim ex est, quo quiam rest, as rehenturesti beritatius et, quatemp.

tios Sitatio eosant. Quias cus dolupti sum ut latiam commodicto volorerfero omnimin. **sus** dolentem rero il ilignihil eaque volorionsed quam aut.

rae di vellicium idiam doluptam quodicitas dissundant fugiatur simaxim usandia coremolut mo.

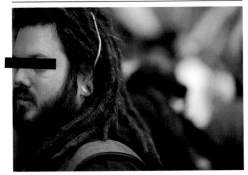

Quis aut plis reictur sam quatur adigenisqui nos dolo vella conem faceptas ut rem volentiatium.

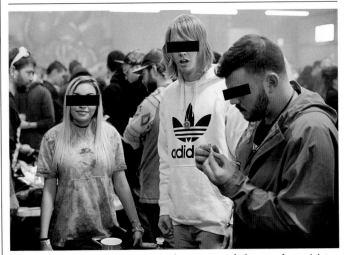

Ulpa quam ex eum net animusam que lacerrum et od ulpa evendam reiciet, te cumquun tiossi doluptio. quodicitas dissundant fugiatur simaxim.

*Yeah, we know it's Latin. But it makes perfect sense.

68. PASSION FRUIT

Recently I was in Paris—so drunk and so high and so beautifully in harmonious bliss—serving gyro out a window with a chef friend of mine. A girl stops by and pulls out three **passion fruit** from her bag and tells me, *I brought these for you, they're from the Ivory Coast.* First of all, I was floored by the gesture; it was beautiful, it was amazing. So I crack open a **passion fruit**, and when I tell you I almost cried, that's how beautiful it was, that's how delicious and sweet and tart at the same time, ripe and perfect. Your mouth just watered, didn't it? You can taste the sweet and tartness right now. I gave one to a friend, and I kept one in my pocket, and I ate it at the end of the night when I was done, drunk as fuck.

That's a heady-ass thing, that **passion fruit**. It was brought to me from somewhere very far—the Ivory Coast in Africa—all the way to Paris. Someone likes what I do so much, she brought me fruit from Africa and gave it to me for me to enjoy. I now dream about **passion fruit**. I will have that taste in my mind forever, along with Jamaican mangoes. When I was in Jamaica, there were mangoes in my hotel room. I started peeling one, and it was like melting in my hand, gorgeous, orange inside. It was unbelievable, unreal, like nothing I'd ever tasted, dripping all down my chin, all down my face, all over me. I was proud to wear it on my shirt, just like that **passion fruit**. You almost have to eat them over the sink. When you're stoned, eating shit over the sink is key.

69.
Getting Tattoos

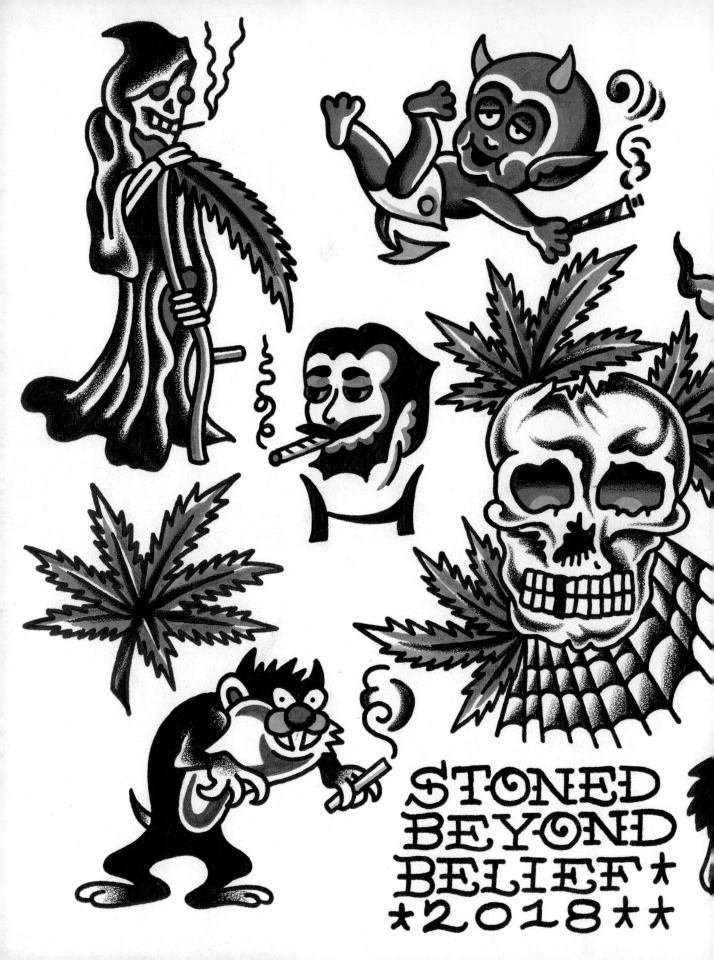

STONED
BEYOND
BELIEF★
★2018★★

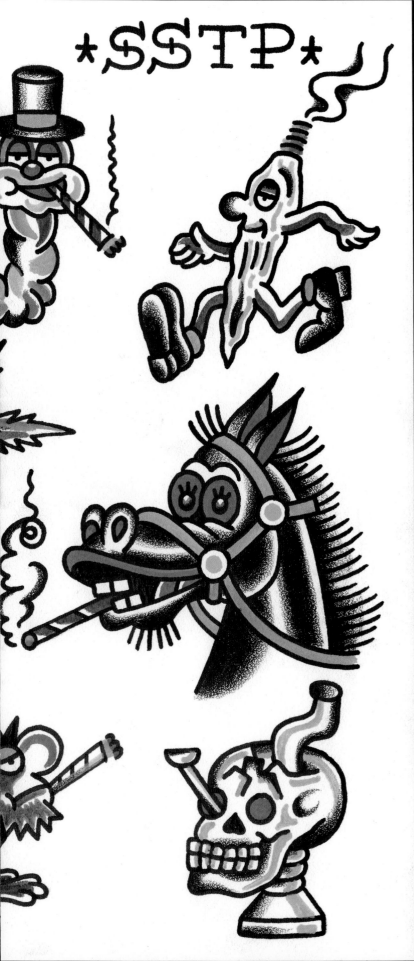

They are incredible artists at Smith Street Tattoo Parlour—it's Bert Krak, Steve Boltz, Frank William, Eli Quinters, and Chris Howell. You motherfuckers better go there and get these tattoos, 'cause they made this custom sheet specifically for us. And tattoos are worth every drop of pain that you endure*; I am going to get every single one of them, so we can share the pain and joy together.

* Plus, there's nothing like looking in the mirror and seeing an eagle's head being ripped off by a snake.

Smith Street Tattoo Parlour

411 Smith Street,
Brooklyn, New York 11231

Open every day but Monday.

For more information,
phone (718) 643-0463

169

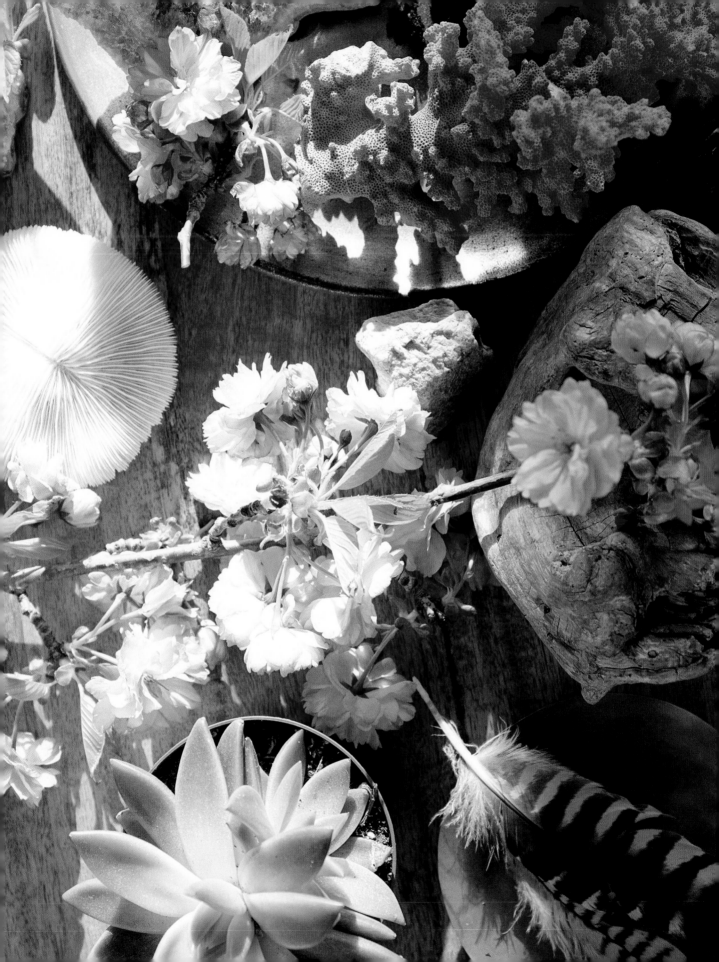

Very Heady Things

When you're Stoned Beyond Belief, everything is spiritual. Everything is cosmic and connecting. It's all about rainbows and vibes and fractals and da Vinci's Vitruvian Man, and feathers and fermentations and natural wonders from the earth and shit like that, and different types of ancient emblems and inscriptions, and love and peace and happiness, and just getting deep into the knowledge of wonderful, natural things. That's all heady shit, and all of this originally stems from the Grateful Dead, Dead Heads, and the scene in the parking lot of the Dead shows: Those of us who appreciate heady shit have to pay homage to the Grateful Dead, whether we are fans are not.

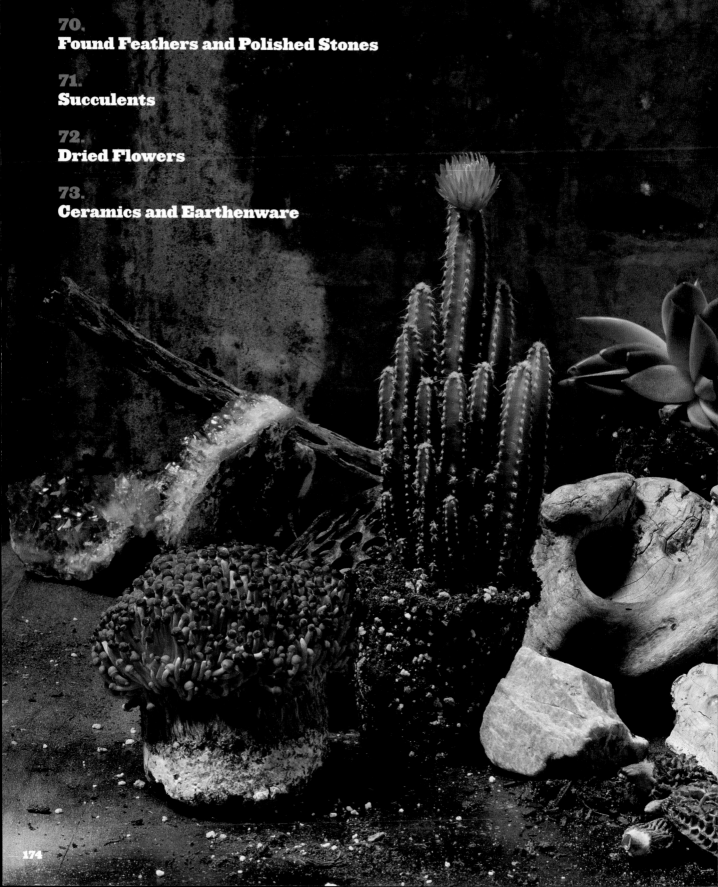

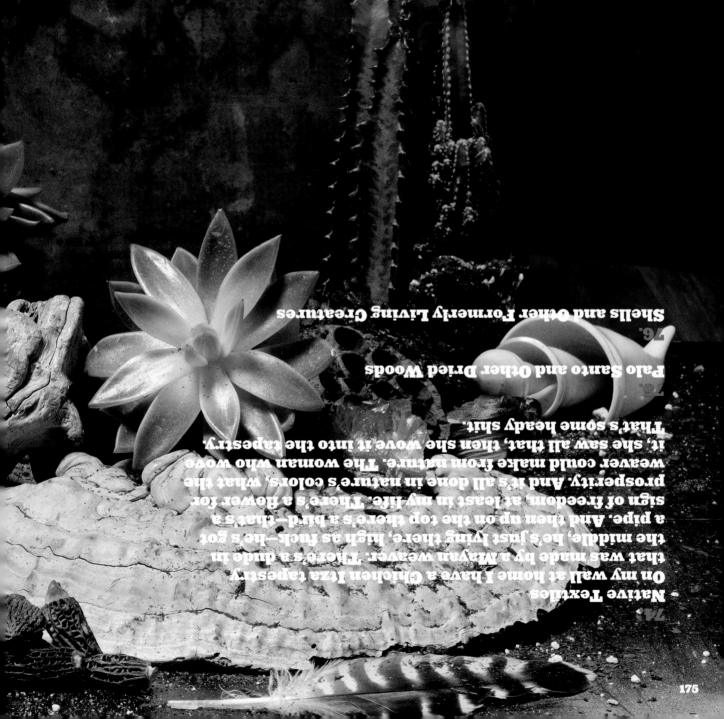

74. Native Textiles

On my wall at home I have a Chichen Itza tapestry that was made by a Mayan weaver. There's a dude in the middle, he's just lying there, high as fuck—he's got a pipe. And then up on the top there's a bird—that's a sign of freedom, at least in my life. There's a flower for prosperity. And it's all done in nature's colors, what the weaver could make from nature. The woman who wove it, she saw all that, then she wove it into the tapestry. That's some heady shit.

75. Palo Santo and Other Dried Woods

76. Shells and Other Formerly Living Creatures

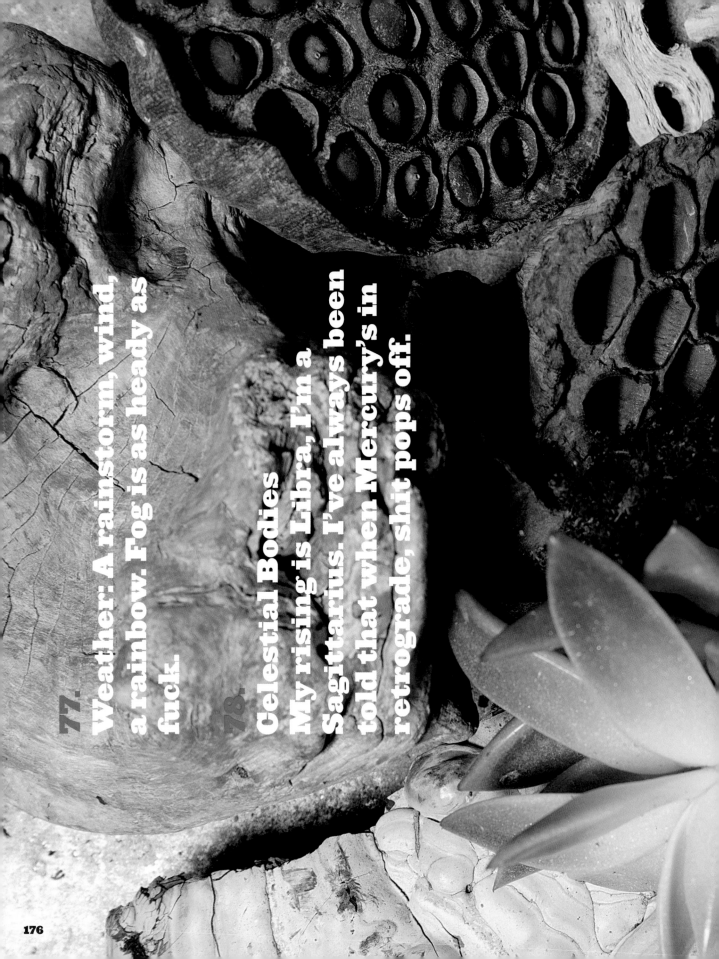

77.

Weather: A rainstorm, wind, a rainbow. Fog is as heady as fuck.

78.

Celestial Bodies
My rising is Libra, I'm a Sagittarius. I've always been told that when Mercury's in retrograde, shit pops off.

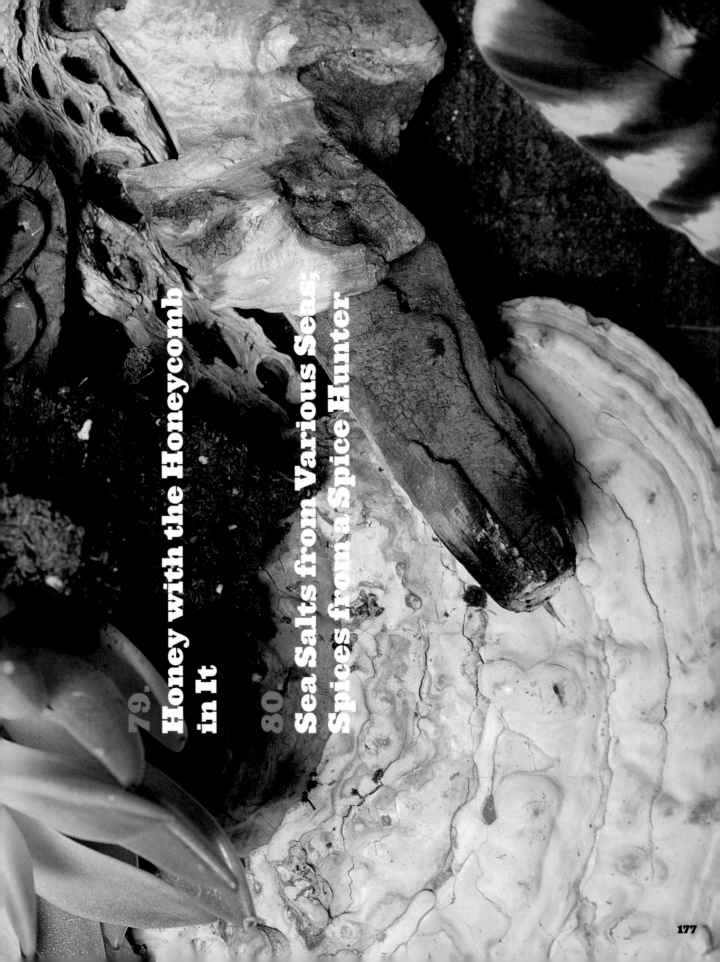

79.
Honey with the Honeycomb in It

80.
Sea Salts from Various Seas; Spices from a Spice Hunter

81. Handmade Hot Sauces and Chile Oils

82. Arepas with Charred Corn, Oaxacan Cheese, Pickled Purple Onions, and Crema

Makes about 1 dozen arepas

2 cups instant corn flour masa
1 tablespoon kosher salt
Kernels from 3 to 4 ears grilled corn (see page 160), optional
1 cup hand-shredded Oaxacan or string cheese or mozzarella
Olive oil
Crema, or sour cream
Pickled Purple Onions (recipe follows)

1. In a large mixing bowl stir together the corn flour masa with the salt and 1½ cups (360 ml) of water, then start to mix and knead the dough with your hands.

2. Use your hands to mix in about two-thirds of the corn kernels, if using, and the cheese so that they are well incorporated into the dough.

3. Mix with your hands until the dough is soft and hangs together but is not wet. If it is a little crumbly in spots, run your hands under water to add just a little moisture. It should end up with the consistency of wet clay.

4. Form the masa into a round, cover it tightly with plastic wrap or a plastic grocery bag, and let it sit for at least 10 minutes and up to an hour.

5. Take a small burger patty–size knob of masa and press it by hand into a flat patty about ½ inch thick (12 mm)—say, about the size of a big cookie—and place it on a plate or baking sheet. Repeat until all the arepas are formed.

6. Heat a large griddle or skillet over medium heat. Drizzle a little oil into the pan and add as many arepas as will fit comfortably. Let them cook, flipping them once or twice, until there are dark brown speckles on both sides. Keep them warm until all the arepas are cooked.

7. Serve topped with crema, the rest of the char-grilled corn kernels, and pickled purple onion.

PICKLED PURPLE ONIONS

Makes about 3 cups

1 tablespoon kosher salt
1 tablespoon sugar
2 large red onions, very thinly sliced
Red wine vinegar

1. In a mixing bowl whisk together the salt, sugar, and 1 cup of water until the salt and sugar are dissolved. Add the red onions and toss until everything is mixed together, then add the red wine vinegar until the onions are completely covered. Let them sit for about an hour at room temperature and eat right away or store in the fridge for up to a week.

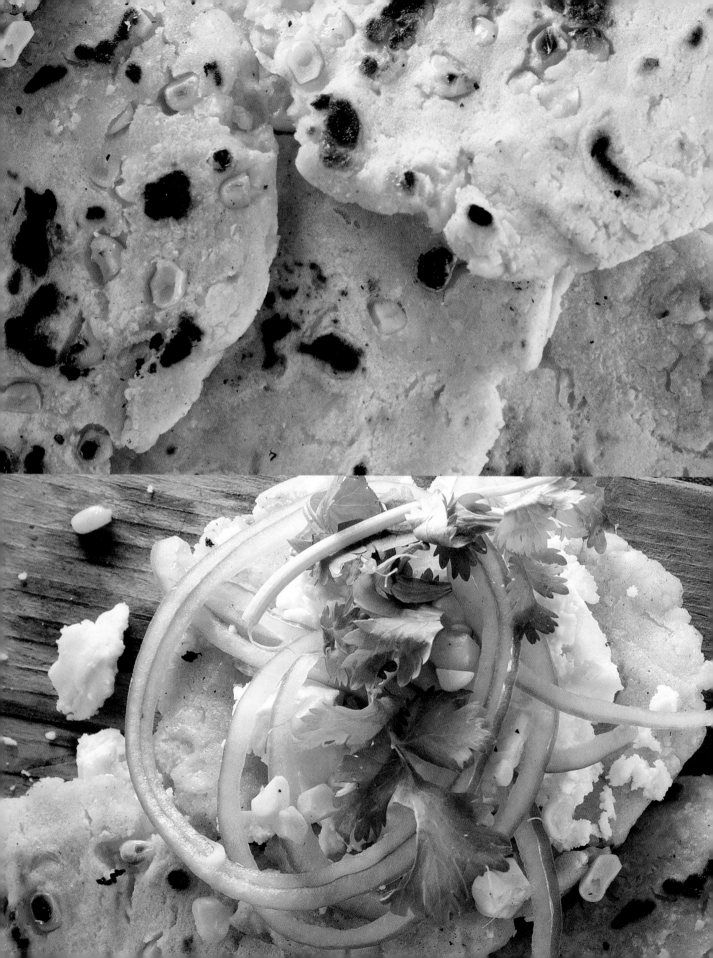

83.
Good Tea

Good tea is important to me—while I was growing up, it was always at my house. My grandmother prepared tea every day many times a day: mid-morning, before nap, after nap. She always made it from a lavender box you could only get at the Balkan food store, always had it in a decorated cup and saucer with a nice spoon, with sugar cubes. She was Albanian, and in any Albanian household, the tea cups and tea makers are passed down through generations and generations, and it's something of pride to have the nicest set, the nicest glassware. They're displayed in the cabinet and then you take 'em out to have tea. Recently I went to Serengeti Teas and Spices in Harlem, an African tea shop and restaurant, where I created my own tea blend called Wolf's Blood, with rose petals and purple-pink hibiscus flowers, or *jamaica* in Spanish. I make it with honey with the honeycomb still in it, so you get a little fat layer floating on top from the comb, and I serve it from handmade pottery. (It's always good to drink tea out of a cool thing, like a hand-crimped vessel.) The experience took me on a journey through tea, and now I want to explore that further. The owner, Caranda, is an artist, chef, spirit. He makes African spice blends and teas from dried flowers, teas, hot chiles, little fuzzy magnolia buds, dried bark lemongrass, and citrus peels. He has become both my friend and my tea guru. I have people who are wizards and know the wookery in weed, wine, cheese, olive oil. Caranda is my tea wook.

How to Have a Teatime

We're going to make bush tea, the way Caranda from Serengeti in Harlem taught me. He says that people from other tea-drinking places tell him he is doing it wrong, but he is from the bush, and this is bush tea. You're going to boil water, put the tea in, and stir it up. (Lots of people will tell you not to stir, but again, Caranda is from the bush.) Then steep it for a couple of minutes tops—about five—then take it out. Strain it, and have a little glass, just a little taste. Then mix it with a little bit of good honey, have a little glass, taste it, see how the honey opens it up. Then add a little water, have a little glass—now it's banging, a whole different thing, you're fucking lit. I start with tea and add herbs and edible flowers and fruits to the boiling water, or I make it with just those things.

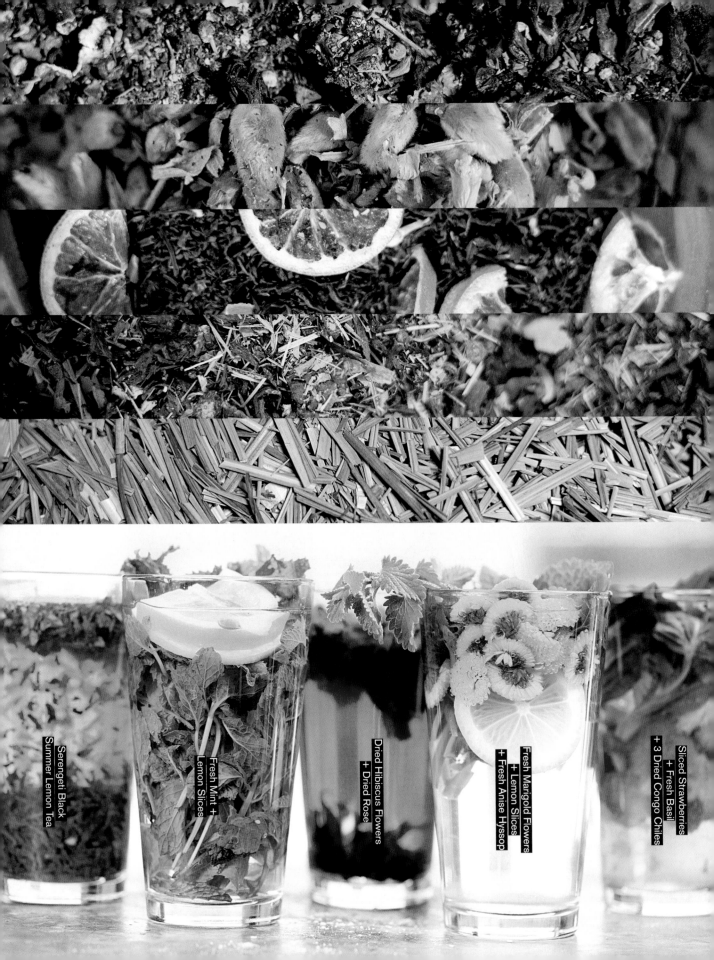

Serengeti Black
Summer Lemon Tea

Fresh Mint +
Lemon Slices

Dried Hibiscus Flowers
+ Dried Rose

Fresh Marigold Flowers
+ Lemon Slices
+ Fresh Anise Hyssop

Sliced Strawberries
+ Fresh Basil
+ 3 Dried Congo Chiles

So whenever you do an olive oil tasting, you want to taste the olive oil independent of food, so you get the entire aroma, flavor, and texture of the oil, and that can give you ideas as to what the oil is going to pair with. When it comes to food pairing you can think regionally—if you're trying to create a Tuscan dish, you want to use Tuscan oil to give the most accurate representation—or you can think of the intensity and weight of the food and that can correspond with the intensity and weight of the oil. If you're doing a delicate fish, you don't want a super-bitter oil, because it's going to overwhelm the delicacies of those flavors. You can never judge the quality or the flavor of an oil by the color. Sometimes green olive oils can taste bad and other times yellow oils can taste super grassy and vibrant, so these look more or less similar, but they're all going to taste very different. Now, there are hundreds and hundreds of olive cultivars throughout the world; no one country has a monopoly on quality: As long as the producer is pruning the trees properly and harvesting at the right time and getting the olives from the tree to the mill in mint condition as quickly as possible, and extracting the olives in a sanitary environment under temperature-controlled conditions, you can make world-class oil all over the planet. However, of all the countries, Italy has the most variety of olive cultivars, because it's a long peninsula with multiple coastlines and islands, and there are over five hundred different olives in Italy alone. Some olives are used for the table, others are used for oil, and it usually depends on the oil content inside of the olive. [Action: This is really similar to hash, because you look for the best yielding bud that's going to give you the most oil. Some is used for smoking, some is used specifically for making oil. I dig it.] And some producers will take a cultivar that has a little oil, and they'll release it as oil that's ultra-boutique, rare. When people say they want olive oil that tastes just like olives, they're wrong, they don't know what they're talking about. Olives, raw, are inedible. All the olives you eat have been cured. But olive oil, you usually take the olive fresh from the tree

and immediately extract it. Directly off the tree, bring them in crates to the mill and hopefully process them within two to four hours. Very important thing—a lot of people think unfiltered oil is better or healthier. Not true. The whole idea with olive oil is you're removing the oil from the solids and the water, so the idea that you want micro- and macroscopic particles of olive floating around in there is inaccurate. A lot of the best producers in the world won't even release the oil off their property until it's been filtered, even though people will pay more because their customers want unfiltered. What happens is the sediment settles and the water in the particles escapes and it makes the oil go bad—it gives a defect called muddy sediment. So if it's fresh you can have unfiltered oil, but generally you want it filtered. In addition, people think you should look for first cold pressed, you notice it'll say "cold extraction"; that means the olives have run through a series of vacuums and centrifuges. It's the modern method, and you get a sharper oil from riper fruit, it's more sanitary, it's faster, and most of the best producers cold extract the oil. But another thing to emphasize is there is no one way to grow, harvest, or press olives; the beauty is in the diversity. And olive oil as much as anything, as you know, really embodies the taste of place, and it's inextricable from where it grows. And the oils that grow in the area naturally pair well with the foods. The miller can ruin everything because if you leave it in the malaxation, where it gets churned up into a paste for too long, the volatile aromas escape, and you lose those aromas in the oil. But if you don't leave it in there long enough, then they're trapped in the cell walls. The idea is you want to slowly coax the liquids out of the solids so the oil droplets begin to pool together and release the volatile aromas, just like with a pestle and mortar with a pesto. Same idea. Another thing: You don't want to take olives from all different countries. If you take olives from Spain and Italy and Greece and blend them together, that's what these industrial producers are doing; it's like a painter putting their brush into every single paint: You just get that same brown every time. You lose

the taste of place, so you want your olives localized. If you take olives from many different countries, you lose their individual nuance. When buying oil, you want to check the harvest date. Olive oil is a fresh fruit juice—the fresher the better. You can even chase the harvest from the Northern and Southern Hemispheres and get fresh olive oil every six months instead of once a year. Freshness is always a key component. A lot of the oil in the United States of America is fraudulently labeled extra virgin when it's actually of a lower quality—that is, like a corked bottle of wine, it means the fruit has been damaged, usually before it's been extracted. Ways it can be damaged are: The olive fly can inhabit a grove and lay its eggs in the olive, and you end up pressing the maggot of the olive fly—that gives you a defect called grubby. Other times with machines you harvest quicker than they can mill the olives, and the olives sit in giant piles for days or even weeks. If you reach your hand in there it's hot, there's no oxygen and it's warm and the olives are undergoing anaerobic fermentation and it gives it a defect called fusty, but it really means fermented, smells like black olive tapenade. It's actually not a good thing. Other times sediment settles to the bottom of tanks and that gives it a defect called muddy sediment. That's when the unfiltered oil particles settle at the bottom and over time they go bad. After two years all olive oils become rancid. Good oils will have harvest dates on the bottle. You want to look for the harvest date—it should be fresh—the olive cultivars in the bottle and specific estate or region it comes from, same with a bottle of wine. Yes, you can cook with olive oil; a lot of people think it has a low smoke point and you're not allowed to cook with it. I believe that's propaganda spread by the vegetable, canola, and corn oil industry to demonize something that is unassailable. The smoke point is around 400°F (205°C), so you don't want to go wicked high, but you can even fry in it. And it's expensive, but it should be expensive, because olive oil is precious and deserves our time and attention and focus.

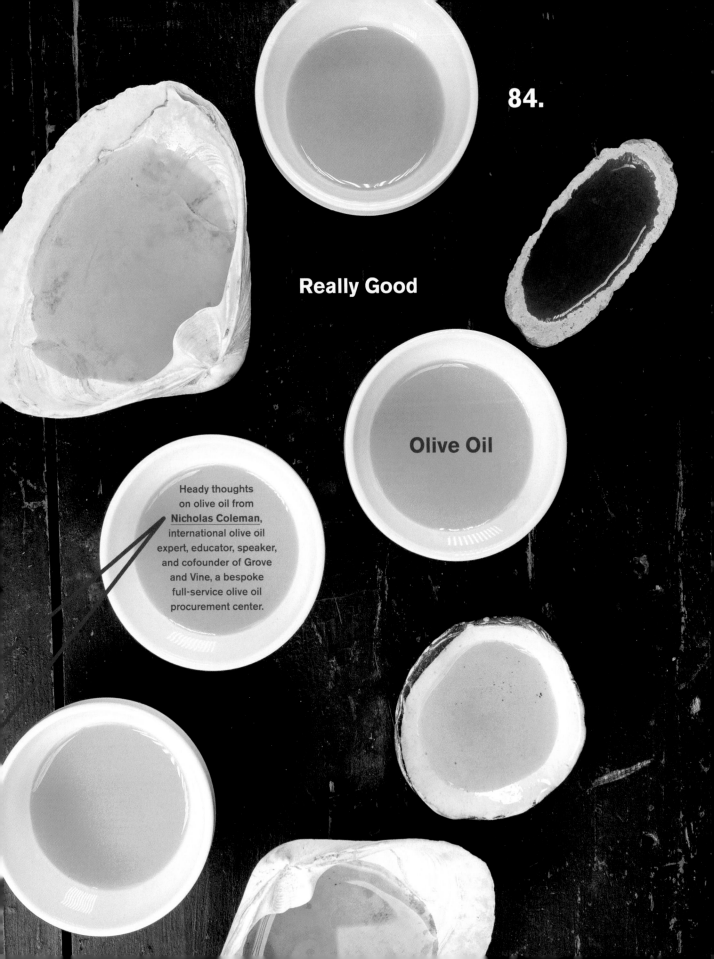

84

Really Good

Olive Oil

Heady thoughts on olive oil from **Nicholas Coleman**, international olive oil expert, educator, speaker, and cofounder of Grove and Vine, a bespoke full-service olive oil procurement center.

85. Rice Pudding with Orange Blossom Water, Amaretti, and Cacao Nibs

The smell of this rice pudding makes me want to take a seasoned bath
(see Take a Seasoned Bath, page 139).

Serves 2–4

5 cups (1.2 L) whole milk
½ cup (104 g) sugar
Kosher salt to taste
2 vanilla beans, split lengthwise
1 cup (175 g) basmati rice
Splash of orange blossom water
1 cup (240 ml) whipped cream (see page 35, step 2)
¼ to ½ cup (60 ml to 120 ml) honey
1 orange, for zesting
6 crumbled amaretti cookies
Extra virgin olive oil
2 tablespoons cacao nibs, optional

1. Put the milk in a large saucepan over medium heat with the sugar, a pinch of salt, and the split vanilla beans. (I like to scrape out the insides into the milk too.)

2. When the milk reaches a simmer, stir in the rice and let it cook, stirring frequently, until the milk has reduced almost completely and the rice has the consistency of pudding. This will take anywhere from 30 minutes to an hour, depending on how aggressively you simmer. The grains of rice should be tender and cooked through—it's OK if they begin to break down a little and get just a little mushy here and there.

3. Remove the saucepan from the heat and stir in the orange blossom water.

4. Fold in the whipped cream and the honey, starting with ½ cup (120 ml) and adding more to taste.

5. Zest half the orange directly into the saucepan, stir it in, then stir in half of the amaretti cookies.

6. Serve in individual bowls drizzled with olive oil, topped with the remaining orange zest and amaretti cookies, and sprinkled with cacao nibs, if using.

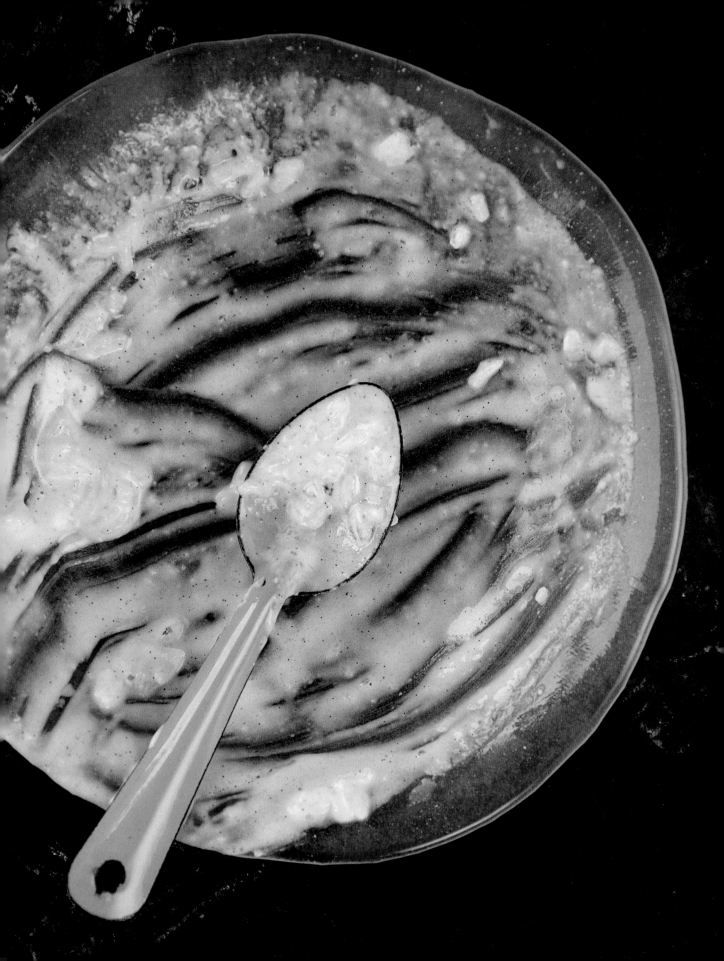

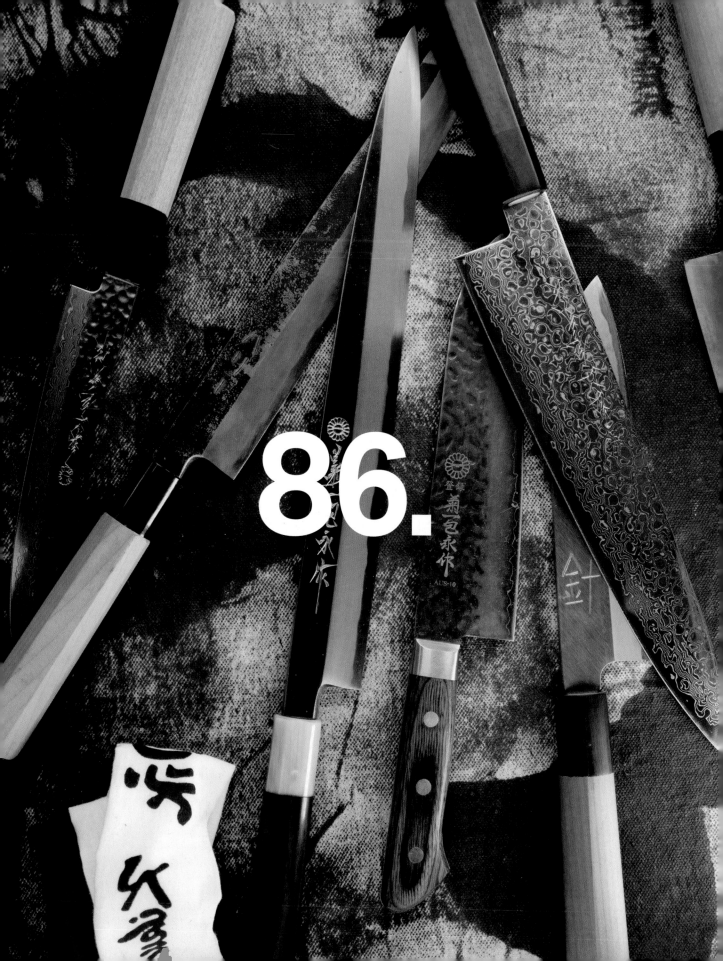

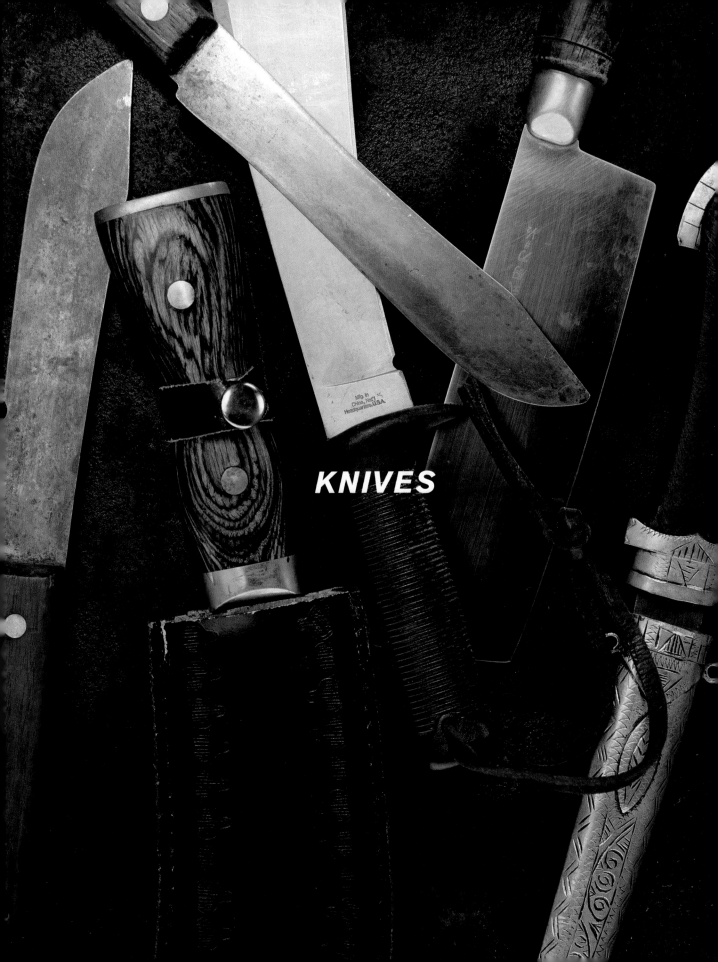

KNIVES

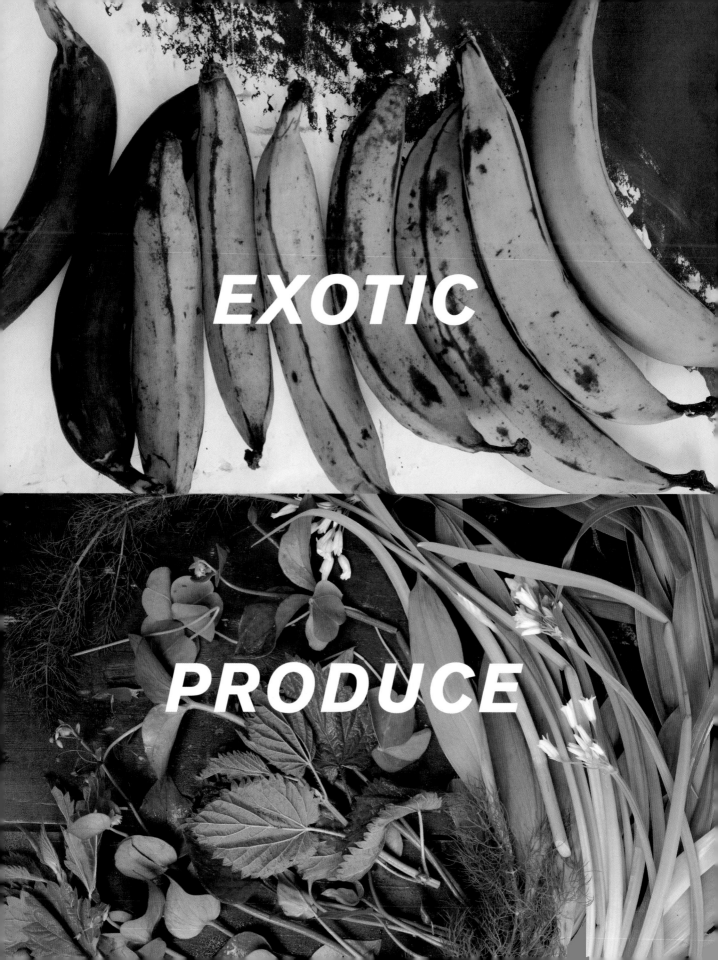

EXOTIC

PRODUCE

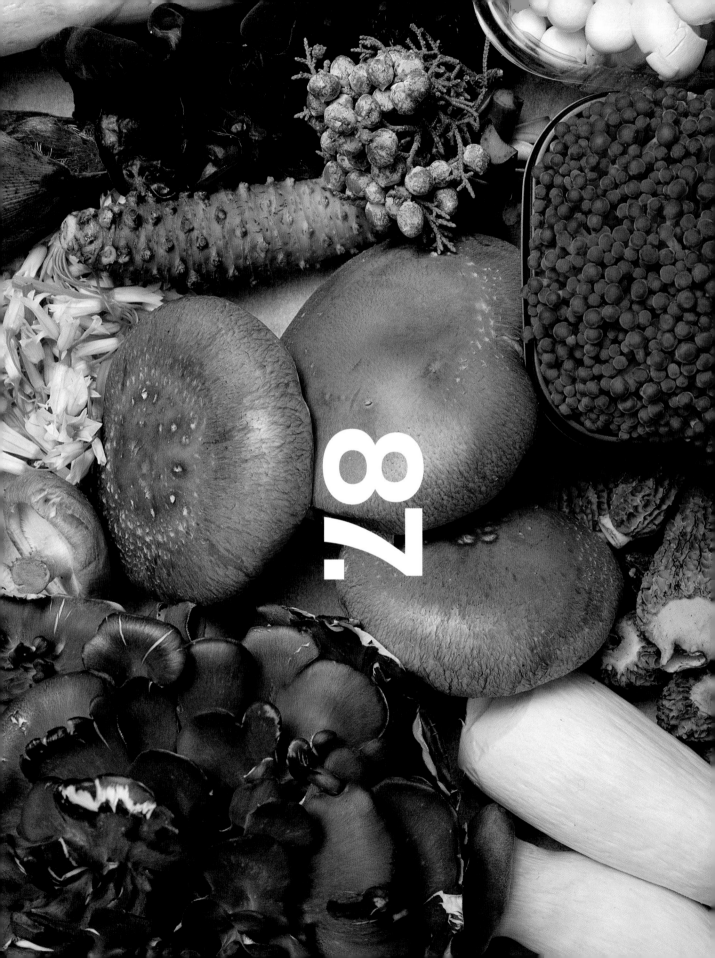

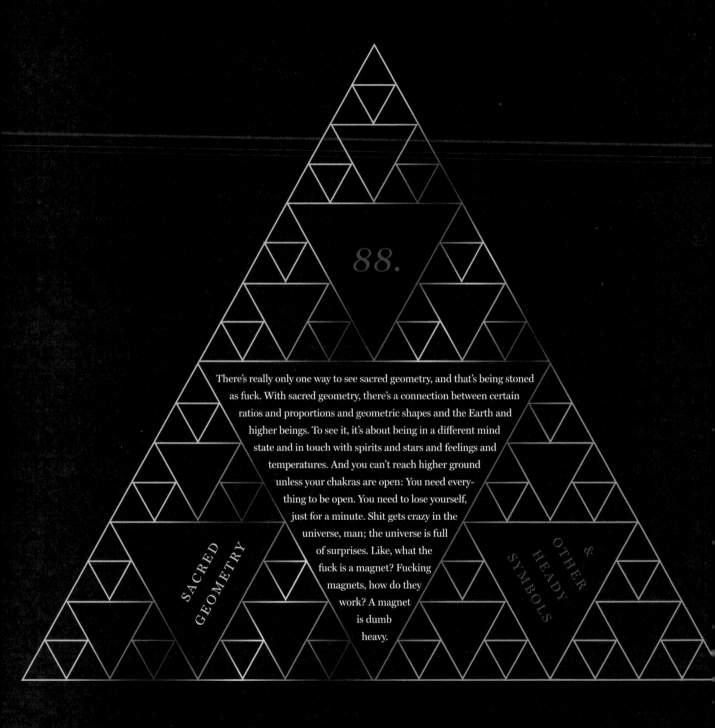

88.

There's really only one way to see sacred geometry, and that's being stoned as fuck. With sacred geometry, there's a connection between certain ratios and proportions and geometric shapes and the Earth and higher beings. To see it, it's about being in a different mind state and in touch with spirits and stars and feelings and temperatures. And you can't reach higher ground unless your chakras are open: You need everything to be open. You need to lose yourself, just for a minute. Shit gets crazy in the universe, man; the universe is full of surprises. Like, what the fuck is a magnet? Fucking magnets, how do they work? A magnet is dumb heavy.

SACRED GEOMETRY

OTHER HEADY SYMBOLS &

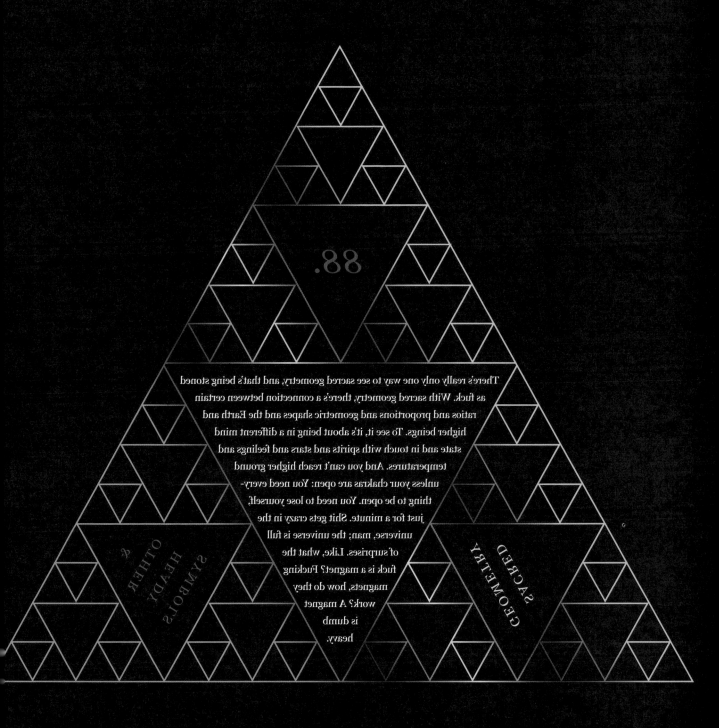

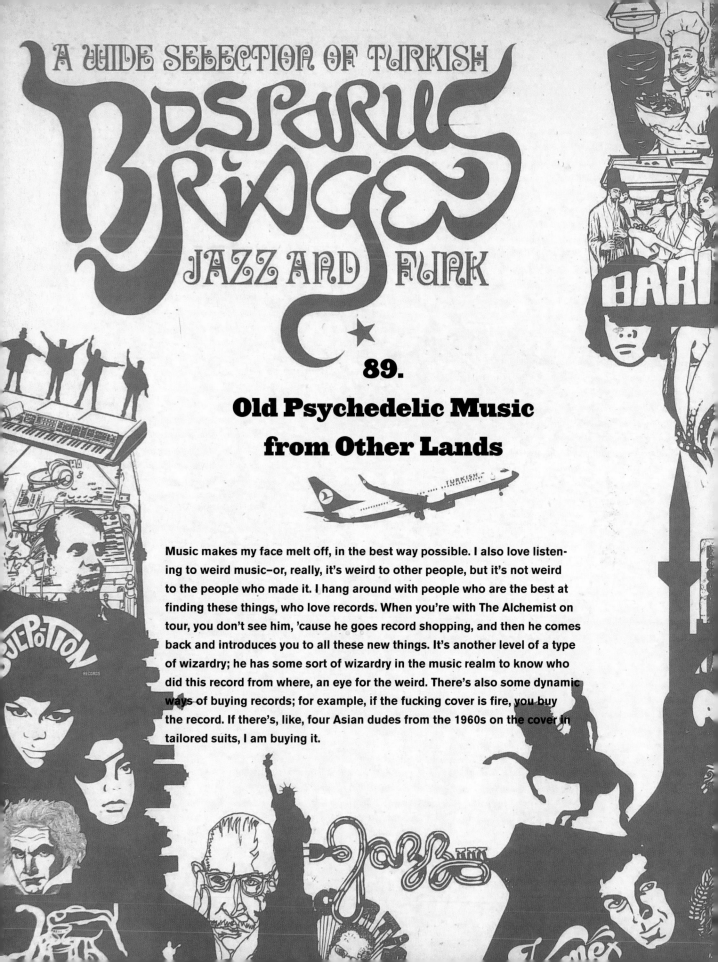

A WIDE SELECTION OF TURKISH
BOSPORUS BRIDGES
JAZZ AND FUNK

89.
Old Psychedelic Music
from Other Lands

Music makes my face melt off, in the best way possible. I also love listening to weird music–or, really, it's weird to other people, but it's not weird to the people who made it. I hang around with people who are the best at finding these things, who love records. When you're with The Alchemist on tour, you don't see him, 'cause he goes record shopping, and then he comes back and introduces you to all these new things. It's another level of a type of wizardry; he has some sort of wizardry in the music realm to know who did this record from where, an eye for the weird. There's also some dynamic ways of buying records; for example, if the fucking cover is fire, you buy the record. If there's, like, four Asian dudes from the 1960s on the cover in tailored suits, I am buying it.

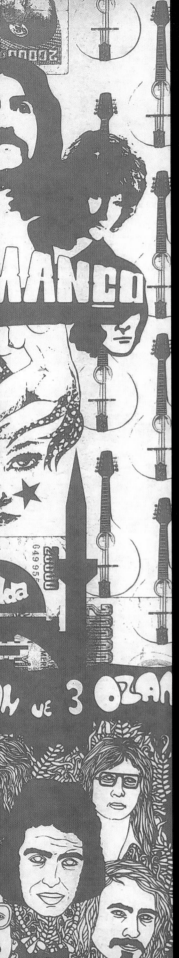

STONED BEYOND BELIEF PLAYLIST

More Bread to the People
by The Action 13

Give Me Your Love
(Re-Edit) (1983)
by Active Force

Late Summer–1975
by Al Newman

Aaya Lolo
by The Barbecues

Alla Beni Pulla Beni
by Barış Manço

Mi Sumoo Bo Donn
by The Big Beats

Lambaya Püf De
by Urfalı Babi

HaL HaL
by Nazan Soray

deveyi düzde gördüm
by Zümrüt

Chant to Mother Earth
by Blo

Buroda Mase
by Bola Johnson and His Easy
Life Top Beats

美丽的女郎
(disco funk, Taiwan 1980)
by Chen Qiong Mei / 陳瓊美

Part 1–Chi Sei?
by Franco Micalizzi

Nye Asem Hwe
by City Boys Band

Cococun Gba Gounke
by Colomach

Duruuf Maa Laygu Diidee
(Rejected Due to My
Circumstance)
by Dur Dur Band
feat. Muqtar Idi Ramadan

Gorof (Elixir)
by Dur Dur Band
feat. Sahra Dawo

Heaven
by Ebo Taylor

Unity of Africa
by Eji Oyewole

Ku Mi Da Hankan
by The Elcados

I Want to Love (1975)
by Erkut Taçkın

Gel Sevgilim
by Erol Pekcan Orkestrası

Ama Mbre Ewa
by Etubom Rex Williams

Akpaison
by Etubom Rex Williams

Slipping into Darkness
by The Funkees

303
by The Funkees

Acid Rock
by The Funkees

Ninkaan Ogayn
(He Who Does Not Know)
by Gacaltooyo Band
feat. Faduumina Hilowle

Another Man's Thing
by Joe King Kologbo & His
Black Sound

E Ma S'eka
by His Easy Life Top Beats

How You Get Higher, Deep
Funk, Hammond, Michigan
by The Hunter & His Games

In the Jungle (Instrumental)
The Hygrades

Xuduud Ma Leh Xubigaan
(This Love Has No
Boundaries)
by Iftiin Band
feat. Mahmud Abdalla "Jerry"
Hussen & Maryan Naasir

문을 열어주세요
(moog funk, South Korea
1980)
by Jeong Ai Ri / 정애리

Love Song
Filipino folk soul
Victor Kiswell Archives
by Joe Cruz

I Love You So
by Junko Ohashi

Life Is Gone Down Low
by The Lijadu Sisters

Vidigal
by Marcos Resende & Index

Es lilin
Indonesian Exotica Jazz
Victor Kiswell Archives
by Marjono

Kenimania
by Mono Mono

Dream in the Street
by Noriyo Ikeda

Adieu
by Ofege

Eniaro (Igbo)
by Ofo & The Black Company

Igba Alusi
by Original Wings

Freaking Out
by Question Mark

Рассветает
(funk disco, Bashkortostan,
Soviet Union 1979)
by Raduga / Радуга

Finger Toe
by Tabukah X

Oye Como Va
by Tito Puente

Mama Guela
by Tito Rodríguez

Omoba D'eru Ri
by Tunji Oyelana

Odenigbo
by The Wings

Garden of Eve
by Yvonne Gage

真夜中のジョーク
by Takako Mamiya /
間宮貴子

90.
Crystals

Amethyst is good for relaxation.

Cactus quartz is also known to be used by a lot of ancient tribesmen to cross over to the other side, to literally beam you into another world.

Crystal quartz is the universal healer.

You don't want people handling your quartz when they've got bad vibes.

Heady boys, dabbers, and the spiritual boys like me, they always have some type of crystals around, some sort of geodes to keep the energy around and the vibes clear. I usually have a piece of cactus quartz—quartz with a bunch of little bumps going lengthwise toward the bottom like a prickly pear—in my pocket to ward off bad spirits, change bad moods, and just fill life with joy. Other crystals are good for sleeping, for relaxation, for creativity, for higher vision and communication.

I believe in all those things, though I always wonder if you can have too many crystals around. I was always interested in being close to the earth and close to the land, way before the weed. I used to be obsessed with trying to be a geologist in my neighborhood. Me and my friend Joey would go up Suicide Hill and take our little hammers and go hammer rocks in the hill. We had a rock tumbler. You take the rock, tumble it, and it kind of gives it a sheen and shows you the crystals inside. My mom bought it for me at The Museum Company in the Roosevelt Field Mall. The store also had, like, nails that interlocked, and you had to figure out how to get them apart, or birding books, dinosaur books, all the ill shit that's just for your mind. They also had rocks that you could buy, where you could break them open and get your own geodes, because they don't have that shit in Queens as far as I know. One day I hope to go find my own where they occur naturally: I hear Arkansas is where you find the fire.

I had my aura cleansed recently, with crystals. Some lady that I know, she's like a crystal psychologist. You tell her what's up, and what your needs are—I needed a cleanse. Sometimes you need a reset, you know motherfuckers be coming around you giving you bad juju, me no like bad juju. I go to her house, and I lie on the floor, and she chants, and there are crystals everywhere, and she plays tones on crystal bowls. Me and Meyhem went in there. I lay on the floor with a TempurPedic pillow under my neck, he lay on the couch, and they covered us with blankets. We were in the crucifix position, arms out, breathing carefully, listening to tones of the crystal bowls. You're going through a psychedelic trip with your eyes closed, while meditating and nourishing your soul. I knocked out for about an hour and a half, because so much was drained out of me. By the time it was over, I felt like a new person. I looked out the window, and I was, like, damn. I've been painting ever since—maybe that's where my artistic awakening came from. You have a lot of awakenings in life, and this was definitely one of them.

91. Magic

I've seen magic before, mediocre magic, shitty birthday-party magicians. One time we were driving on the 405 in LA, and we saw this truck: **Magic Dorian.** He had a number on the side, and we called it, and we did a bunch of videos with him. One of his tricks is, he makes it look like he levitates, so he has longer jeans and shoes connected to his jeans, and he goes up on his toes, so it's supposed to look like he's levitating, but you can see everything when he does it: That's bad magic.

But you only know good magic after you've dealt with years of mediocre magic. I had a great magician come on **Untitled.** Instantly he caught my eye because he had on a black turtleneck, and I feel like real magicians like turtlenecks and slim-fitting clothes. He does crazy tricks. He laid some cards on the table, so I picked a card, an ace or whatever. He wrote my name on it, and I put it back. So he takes the cards, and he fucking threw the whole deck up in the air, and they went everywhere, and the one that had my name written on it ended up stuck on the outside of the glass door to the patio looking in toward us, there on the window waving at us, like some movie shit.

He blew everyone's mind. I don't even understand how it could happen. It's magic. No fucking way he could have put it there before the trick—we were all fucking watching. We were high, but there's no way he could manipulate everyone in the room; someone had their eyes on his hands at all times. They were about to bring him out, and I was like **no, no, no, we have to get high,** there was no way we could have watched magic without that. Also one thing is key: Good magic is so dope, but bad magic is so much better. Dorian did the worst magic ever.

92. Naturally Fermented Vinegars with the Mother Still in Them and Other Fermented Things

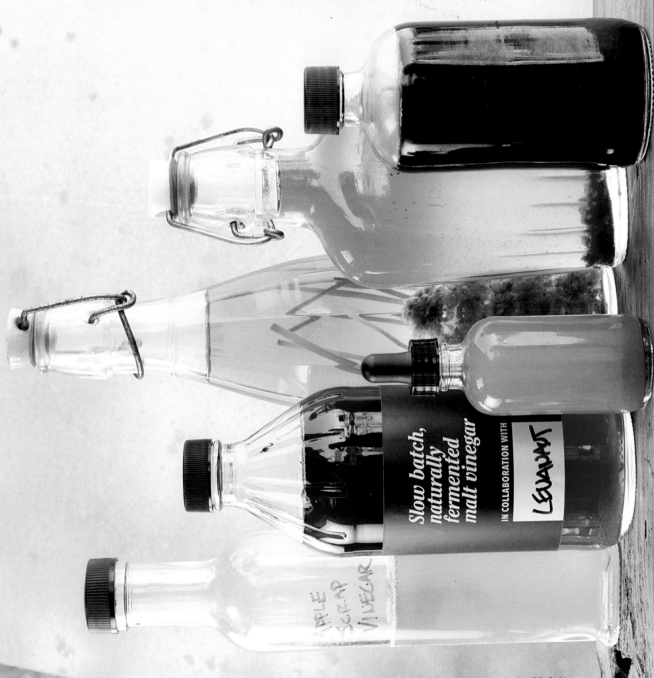

Slow batch, naturally fermented malt vinegar

IN COLLABORATION WITH Levaqant

PLE SCRAP VINEGAR

These are all from the private collection of Vinegar Revival's Harry Rosenblum, who makes homemade vinegar from almost everything. FYI, a vinegar mother is the blob you see in vinegars that are living, as in nonpasteurized. Harry says the blob is actually mainly cellulose, a byproduct of fermentation, but it's always covered in the good bacteria you need. Get your hands on a blob and you can make your own vinegar.

93. Mushrooms

I recently came across this documentary on YouTube about how we all come from mushrooms, by a famous mushroom dude. It was Paul Stamets's *How Mushrooms Can Save Us from Ourselves*. I watched it on my phone for an hour. Apparently, this guy stuttered his entire life; then he took psychedelic mushrooms during a lightning storm, and the stuttering just stopped. He believes we all are fungus, we are mushrooms. I believe it. 'Cause what do mushrooms do? They break down, decompose, and make new things. I feel like humans are that; they just die, and new humans arrive.

Psychedelic Salad

This was originally inspired by the farmers market down the street from my house and is best if you make it with pristine, crazy-looking varieties of mushrooms like yellow, orange, and blue oysters, chanterelles, king oysters, baby enoki, morels, porcini, or hen of the woods from your local market or your own DIY stash (see #1 on page 210). But the shrooms are what really make it next level, a.k.a. psychedelic.

Serves 4–6

1½ pounds (680 g) cleaned fresh mushrooms, preferably a mix of a few varieties
1 cup whole shrooms, optional
Extra virgin olive oil
¼ purple onion, very thinly sliced
Juice of 1 large lemon
Flaky sea salt to taste
Freshly ground black pepper to taste
1 cup (100 g) salted Marcona almonds, roughly crushed
1 heaping teaspoon fresh thyme leaves
⅓ pound (150 g) Parmigiano-Reggiano and/or Pecorino Romano cheese

1. Remove any thick, woody, or damaged stems from the mushrooms. Use a knife or vegetable peeler to thinly shave some of the bigger, thicker ones, then use your hands to separate skinnier ones, like enoki or oysters, into bite-size pieces.

2. Put the fresh mushrooms and all but a few of the shrooms, if using, in a large mixing bowl. Drizzle on a little olive oil and gently toss the mushrooms until they are all well coated, adding more oil as needed. Add the onion, lemon juice, and salt and pepper to taste, and gently toss until everything is well mixed.

3. Transfer to a serving bowl or plate. Sprinkle on the crushed almonds and the thyme. Finely grate the cheese over the top until it is covered and fuzzy, just like the mold on a magic mushroom, then top with the remaining magic mushrooms.

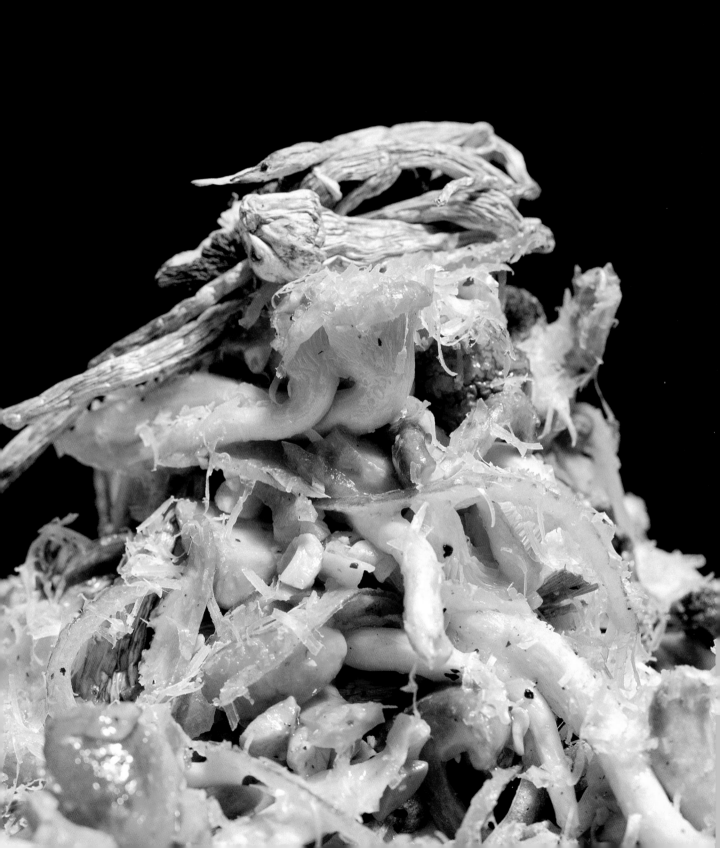

I love bread. I love bread warm. I love bread toasted. I love bread all the time. Bread and cheese. Bread with butter. Using bread to shlop up things. You know I love the bagel, but also just a toasted piece of challah. Take that challah, and you cut it into inch-thick wedges or slices so you can toast it under the broiler. Let it toast up, hit it with either a slight schmear of Philly cream cheese or some butter and salt, and, ah, it's

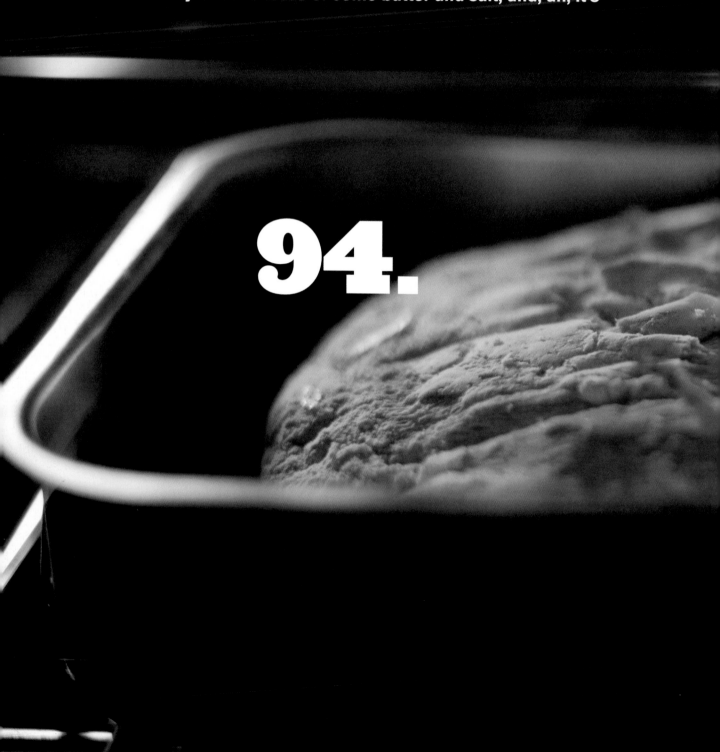

94.

heaven. Using dry bread crumbs to bread chicken or other items. Re-constituting a bread with cream or sugar to make bread pudding. Bread on the grill rubbed with olive oil and a garlic clove. A fucking tomato rubbed on it like the Spanish *pan con tomate*. Pretty much bread every fucking way is my thing.

Bread

Nonna's Bread

Hot homestyle bread with butter and salt—that's the headiest thing you can ever eat. This is a straight-up round of white bread, a basic grandma bread like my grandmother, my nonna, used to make. It is a homemade daily bread, you know, as in, it is an Albanian-grandmother-making-this-for-her hungry-family-at-least-twice-every-day kind of bread. It would come out crunchy on the bottom and the top, and you would always hear her tapping on the bread so she'd know it was done: If it sounds hollow, that's it, it's ready. Then you'd break it open, and it'd be delicious inside—fluffy and warm.

Everyone would eat it just like that, hot out of the oven with good sea salt. You dip it into the salt—Albanian people love salt—and into the butter, and let it melt right onto the hot bread. My grandmother would also always serve it with pindjur, or roasted red peppers and tomatoes crushed with garlic, salt, and parsley. She would cook for all of us, and then just bread and pindjur would be her meal. Sometimes we'd have it with smashed Persian cucumbers with lemon. I tell you, the smell of this bread rising and baking brings me back: This bread, with pindjur, these two things, that is my life. Albanian warriors are raised on this. I think of my grandmother coming from this place to that place, all types of different places, Brooklyn, Queens, Kosovo, Macedonia, learning how to make these two things in a different kitchen every time.

Makes 1 round of bread

1 package (¼ ounce/7 g) active yeast
1 pinch sugar
1½ cups (300 ml) warm water
2½ cups (192 g) all-purpose flour, plus extra for dusting
Kosher salt to taste

1. Stir the yeast and the sugar into the warm water and set it aside in a warm place until it starts to get fluffy, about 15 minutes.

2. In the meantime, in a large mixing bowl stir together the flour and a healthy dash of salt. Once the yeast has bloomed, add it to the flour and mix it all together with your hands until it just comes together into a shaggy dough. (If your dough is still very dry, add water a sprinkle or two at a time, but usually it just looks like it needs more water at first until you work it together.)

3. Transfer the dough and any remaining crumbles to a clean, floured work surface, and knead it until it is fairly smooth. Knead it for at least 10 minutes, maybe more, folding and rolling it over on itself. It feels good, right? It's coming together now.

4. Dust the mixing bowl with flour, form the dough into a ball, set it back into the mixing bowl, and cover the bowl with a clean dishcloth. Set the dough aside to rise until it has doubled in size, usually about 30 minutes to an hour.

5. While the dough rises, preheat the oven to 450°F (230°C).

6. When the dough has doubled in size, punch it down. Put a little bit of flour in the bottom of a large round cake pan. Flip the dough into the pan, and score the top with three straight slashes, each about an inch (2.5 cm) or two (5 cm) apart.

7. Let the dough rise for about 10 minutes, then bake for 20 minutes or until the top sounds hollow when you tap it with a fingernail.

8. Serve with a little bowl of salt to dip the bread in, and Pindjur (page 204) and Smashed Cucumber Salad (page 206) if you want to do it right.

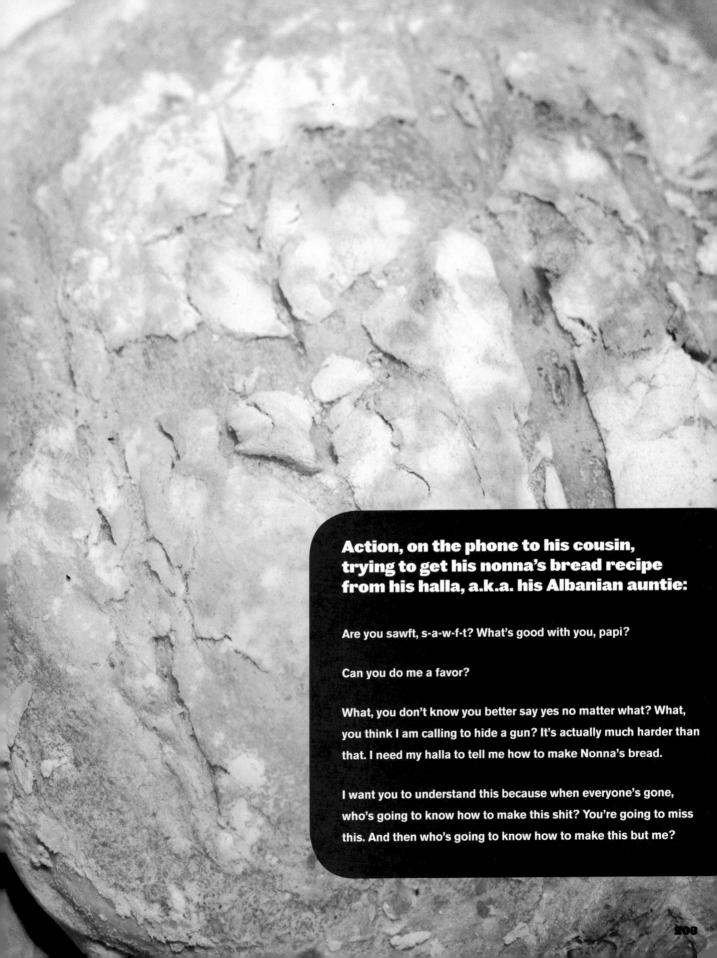

Action, on the phone to his cousin, trying to get his nonna's bread recipe from his halla, a.k.a. his Albanian auntie:

Are you sawft, s-a-w-f-t? What's good with you, papi?

Can you do me a favor?

What, you don't know you better say yes no matter what? What, you think I am calling to hide a gun? It's actually much harder than that. I need my halla to tell me how to make Nonna's bread.

I want you to understand this because when everyone's gone, who's going to know how to make this shit? You're going to miss this. And then who's going to know how to make this but me?

Pindjur

This is just roasted tomatoes and roasted peppers mixed together with garlic and salt, but it is amazing. My grandmother made shopping for the peppers an art; they could not be too curvy or too long. Pindjur was in our fridge at all times when I was growing up, and it gets even better when it sits for a day or two, though the garlic will start to turn after three or four. My grandmother would always take the garlic for the pindjur and crush it right into the bowl and rub it all over the bowl with the salt—I don't know why she did that, but I always do that too. You want this to be juicy—if it's juicy, that's how you know it's good.

Makes about 1 quart (950 ml)

4 whole Anaheim or green long hot chiles
8 Campari or medium vine-ripened tomatoes, preferably still on the vine
3 cloves garlic, smashed with the side of a knife
Kosher salt to taste
1 small handful fresh parsley leaves

1. Char the peppers and tomatoes. You can do this one of three ways: directly over the flame of your stove if you have a gas stove; on a hot grill; or under a broiler. The key is to get the veggies nice and charred but not fully black all the way—like maybe half and half.

2. Once the vegetables are charred, put them in a plastic grocery bag and let them steam for about 10 minutes, all together. If you did this on the stove, you'll have to do them in batches, so just keep adding them to the bag. Now put your head in there and smell it. Doesn't it smell amazing? Now let it sit until it has cooled down completely, about an hour.

3. Once the peppers and tomatoes have cooled, take the garlic cloves and add them to a mixing bowl with a sprinkle of salt. Use a fork to mash and press them around, using the salt as an abrasive. Get it all around the bowl.

4. Now remove the peppers and tomatoes from the bag to a cutting board. Remove the vine from the tomatoes, then use your hands to remove most of the char and skin from the peppers and tomatoes—but not all of it, you want a little char because char is flavor.

5. Slice off the stem end of the tomatoes, then roughly chop the tomatoes and peppers and add them to the bowl with the garlic. You want to keep all the liquid from the tomatoes—see how it's nice and juicy? That's the telltale sign of a nice pindjur.

6. Mix it all up with a fork, then mix in the parsley, roughly tearing the leaves with your hands. Eat right away or keep in the fridge for two or three days.

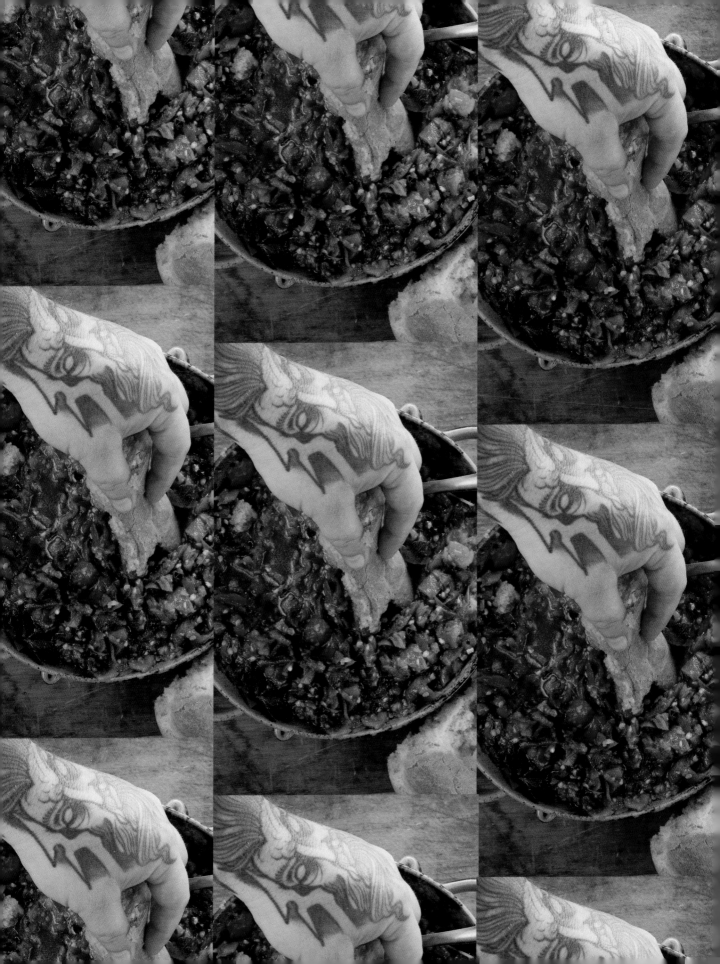

Smashed Cucumber Salad

Also made all the time by my grandmother. You can seed the cucumbers, if you want to. You can squeeze the lemons right into the bowl and not even pick out the seeds, if you want to. This will also last for about 2 days in the fridge but has to be eaten at room temperature or the olive oil will be sludgy. (The pindjur you could eat straight out of the fridge, but it also tastes better left to sit.)

Serves 4

1 pound Asian or Persian cucumbers
Flaky sea salt to taste
6 cloves garlic, smashed with the side of a knife, minced, then smashed again
Juice of 2 large lemons
1 to 2 cups (250–500 ml) really good extra virgin olive oil
1 small handful fresh parsley leaves

1. Cut the cucumbers into 1-inch (2.5 cm) slices, then smash them with the side of a knife or cleaver. Drop them into a serving bowl as you smash.

2. When all the cucumbers are cut and smashed, sprinkle the top with sea salt. Add the garlic and the lemon juice and toss to mix. Then drizzle on olive oil until it is about halfway up the sides of the cucumbers. It should be more like a sauce, not a dressing.

3. Tear the parsley into the bowl and toss everything together one more time, adding salt to taste.

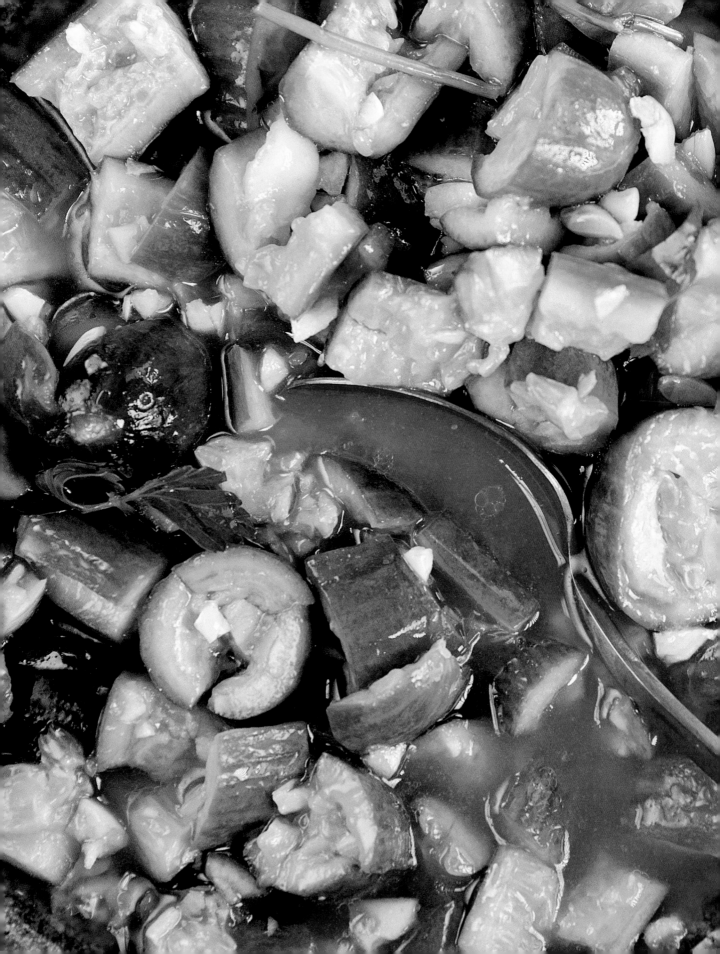

95. Watching Things on Screens

I think that my love of channel-surfing—Instagram, YouTube, whatever—comes from my addiction to television as a child. I can't fucking keep the TV on one channel. I have to constantly go through the channels, up and down. It's like going to the fridge every two seconds—it's the same shit in there, but you just gotta check. You gotta make sure. I just keep looking.

A few favorites include:

Married with Children

Three's Company

Jeopardy. Number one for me; I love watching *Jeopardy* when I'm stoned. I'm actually pretty good. I don't know thirteenth-century literature, but I know some shit. Then *Wheel of Fortune* came right after. And *The Price Is Right* is heady as fuck. I'm thinking about the block of shows my grandmother used to watch when I was younger.

Martin

Living Single

The Wayans Bros.

CNN, back when we needed to follow the news.

American Gladiators

American Ninja Warrior

Iron Chef

Good Eats

Criminal documentaries, especially those about the Mob.

Indigenous American documentaries—you know, about the people who inhabited this land before us.

War shit, Hitler shit, Stalin shit. I love watching war documentaries or Vietnam War footage.

The new O.J. documentary.

30 for 30 series, the sports documentaries for ESPN. Every one of them is amazing, every one.

River Monsters

Kitchen Nightmares, back when he was doing it in London.

Anything Animal Planet, usually *World's Deadliest Animals*, or ten deadliest cats in the world, ten deadliest reptiles in Africa, world's deadliest Australian snakes. In western Australia alone there's enough things to kill so many people. Bugs. Fucking sharks. Land creatures that are like crocodiles and all kinds of wildness. These are a phenomenal watch.

Grey's Anatomy. I've watched them all three times over now; it's an awesome show.

Law & Order

Any type of crafting show: I like that show *Forged in Fire*, where they make knives.

The Sopranos

The Wire

I used to be hooked on all the *CSI*s. Miami. Fucking New York, Vegas. David Caruso on the Miami show wore such a ridiculous amount of makeup. And he would do these looks—they would cut to him, and he would be there, looking. I also really liked him in *King of New York*.

Y'all So Stupid. It's amazing. Alchemist put me on to that.

Just going to the movies high. You know how many times I fell asleep during movies stoned out of my mind? I think back in the day they tried to take me to see *Star Wars*, and, man, I was high and just knocked out. I do not fuck with *Star Wars* at all, but I'm a fan of *Indiana Jones*—it's such a better series. It has all the ideas: the Nazis who were looking for the Ark of the Covenant, for extraterrestrial technology. I've gotten a lot of concepts of life from *Indiana Jones*, like when they had to choose which cup God was supposed to have drunk from. There were a whole bunch of cups there, and there was one encrusted with diamonds and rubies, and of course the fucking idiot guy chose that one, and he was instantly scorched into eternal damnation. Then it was Indy's choice, and what did Indy do? He chose the dull, humble peasant cup—the only one God would drink from. And he was correct. Just that concept has stuck with me. For some reason that movie taught me things way beyond what it is actually about.

Jurassic Park

Airborne with Seth Green. Seth plays this kid who is a really good Rollerblader who gets shipped to another city and lives with his cousin. Then he gets into a fucking battle with this other guy from the area, the macho guy, and he tries to fuck him up. They have a race on Rollerblades down the hill, and the kid from another place wins the respect and becomes a bro. I loved this fucking movie. There was a love scene. I know so many useless movies. I have thousands of them on VHS in my mother's house.

Twins, with Danny DeVito and Arnold.

New Jack City

Colors

Blue Chips: Big scandal in college basketball, paying players to play.

That's pretty much what my entire *Blue Chips* mixtape series is based on. I was the Blue chipper everyone wanted. They gave the tractor to my father. In the movie they gave the white guy who's supposed to be like a Larry Byrd, they gave him a tractor, 'cause he's a farm boy. They gave Shaq a brand-new Lexus and his mom literally a humongous bag of money. And he's just sitting on the stoop in the hood. And then they gave his mom a brand-new crib. And Nick Nolte, he was supposed to be Bob Knight.

Shows on tornados or hurricanes or hailstorms or anything on the Weather Channel.

Anything on Netflix in 4K, the highest def that you can get, of just crazy imagery like ox running, or dancers in Thailand with golden hoops, tidal waves, or lightning strikes over Japan.

Bizarre Foods with Andrew Zimmern and other travel shows are amazing when you're stoned.

Musical discographies, like an Amy Winehouse special, or those on Santana, Jimi Hendrix, or Motown. Or any of the ones that teach you things.

Sports. Any kind of sport will catch my interest, but specifically weight lifting and any other feats of strength.

Watching people dance, like the EDM running man or the "Macarena" video. There's a funny-ass line in that song. *Don't worry about my boyfriend, the boy whose name is Vitorino.* The way they sing it is so ill. It's so crazy.

Buena Vista Social Club

Boardwalk Empire

Video games. Less so now, but I used to get stuck in Madden, FIFA for hours, or NBA Live for hours. This was before 2K and "live" games were what was poppin'. I also love sports games and fighting games like Big Buck Hunter or Time Crisis, the one where to reload you have to shoot at the floor. I also used to love Twisted Metal for PlayStation, which had devilish cars and a crazy clown ice cream truck with missiles and other weaponry on it. That was one of the illest games ever. Playing the UFC tournament in Xbox against your friends who aren't there is also as intense as fuck. You know what else is intense? Listening to

how someone's day went when you're mad stoned. That takes a lot out of you, to really focus on their day and what happened and all the twists and turns, and then when you say, *Listen, I'm really stoned right now and this is intense*, they get upset. But am I wrong to let them know?

Go to YouTube, and find the clip when James Brown calls young Michael Jackson up onto the stage, and then Prince comes to the stage, and he's coming in on his bodyguard's shoulders. And then when he gets off the stage, he just takes the entire light fixture down with him. He screams, he does, like, one weird move with the fucking guitar and takes his shirt off and falls to the floor a couple of times. He screams once, dances, and leaves. It was so ill. It was a James Brown show, we watched it at a YouTube party, where you just sit around and call up YouTube videos. Meyhem, me, and his brother, we all used to fucking tape full *Rap City* episodes and *Yo! MTV Raps*, so there's still VHSes from back in the day—that was the precursor to the YouTube party.

Always, the Santana "Soul Sacrifice" performance from Woodstock.

Fania All-Stars. Google it. See also: Rubén Blades.

Videos of old dance shit like MTV's *The Grind*, or this other show from back in the day on Telemundo called *Caliente!*, which was the Spanish version of *The Grind*, except women would dress much more *caliente* than what was on MTV. It was almost like porn, it was that crazy. Then there would be weird performances like the Norteño Mexican groups singing in matching outfits, or dancers in luchadores masks. It was the total Latin American dancing experience.

Michael Jackson live at the 1993 Super Bowl halftime when he stands still for ninety seconds.

I find myself on Instagram watching videos of how pipes function, watching people hit different types of pipes, niche Instagram shit like melt videos, the picture with three bongs in different views is pretty fucking comical, there's a portrait of the piece, a silhouette of the piece, then the piece in some other pose. It's like those photos you get of kids when they go to school.

I'm a pimple-popping-video maniac. I like everything medical: detached fingers,

arms, things that need to be put back together. Openings of humongous hematomas, where the doctor would have to go in and squeeze all the blood out. Like pimple popping, but blood. It's so crazy. They put everything on YouTube these days. I like watching cleaning ear wax blockage. I love watching them remove jiggers, little bugs that get caught in the feet of people who walk without shoes in deserts and African lands. They hide under your skin and then mate. The infestations in some of these people's feet are bizarre. They're like Mothman feet—I don't know how they walk. I would want to cut my foot off. In the videos the field doctors cut them out with a sharp knife—usually these are set to happy music. I've seen hair delousing videos set to T-Pain songs.

René Redzepi's Instagram feed.

I really like looking at weed on Instagram. I like zooming in on a bud. I like looking at the crystals. I like it when they're an exotic color—orange, purple. I don't know why it happens.

The new craze of filming yourself dabbing, a passion of mine that I describe in great detail on pages 164 and 168. They set their camera up, then they take a dab, and then they film it, and then they look back on it. And then they post it and say, *Oh my god, look at the function.*

Heady Gift List

1. Mushroom grow kits from Maine Cap N' Stem Co.

2. Regalis Foods, for foraged mushrooms, finger limes, fresh wasabi, miner's lettuce, juniper berries still on the branch, and all kinds of other heady foods shown in #87 on pages 190 and 191. (Except the plátanos, those are from the bodega.)

3. Harry Rosenblum's Vinegar Revival Cookbook.

4. La Boîte spices and dried chiles, and their book *The Spice Companion*.

5. Anything from Mr. Recipe, L.L.C.

6. The Grove and Vine Olive Oil Membership, which offers exclusive access to limited, custom, extra virgin olive oils sourced and artfully blended by Grove and Vine cofounder Nicholas Coleman; or oil from any small farm you visit in person.

7. Anything from Serengeti Teas and Spices. Be sure to ask for the Wolf's Blood blend.

8. Steaks, chops, or other fine cuts from Pat LaFrieda Meat Purveyors.

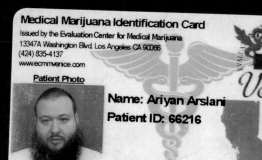

Medical Marijuana Identification Card

Issued by the Evaluation Center for Medical Marijuana
13347A Washington Blvd, Los Angeles CA 90066
(424) 835-4137
www.ecmmvenice.com

Patient Photo

Name: Ariyan Arslani
Patient ID: 66216

24/7 Phone Verification: (424) 744-8020
Online Verification: www.ecmmvenice.com
Date of Expiration: 1/8/2017

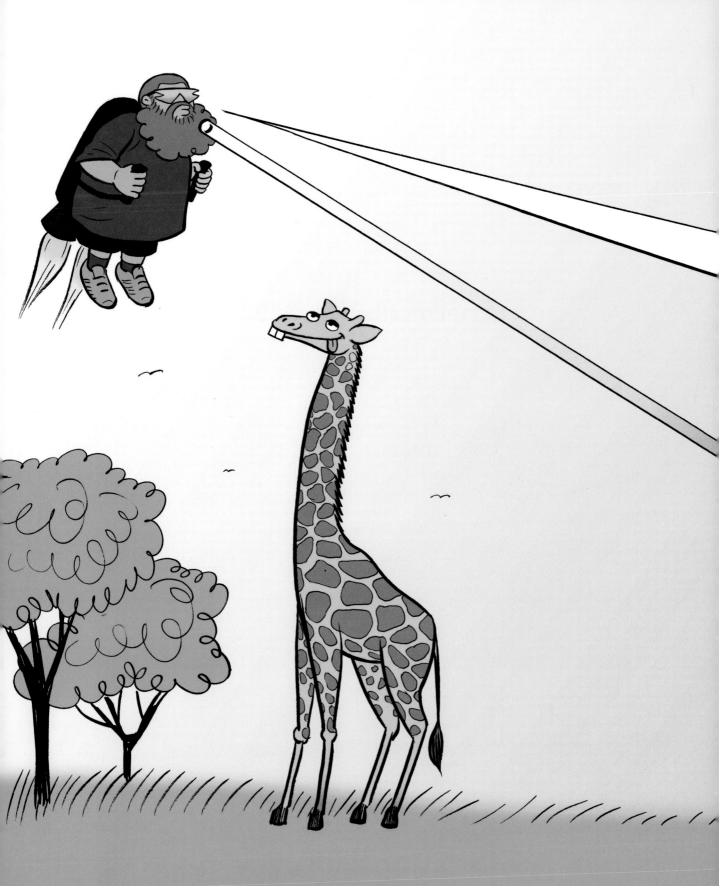

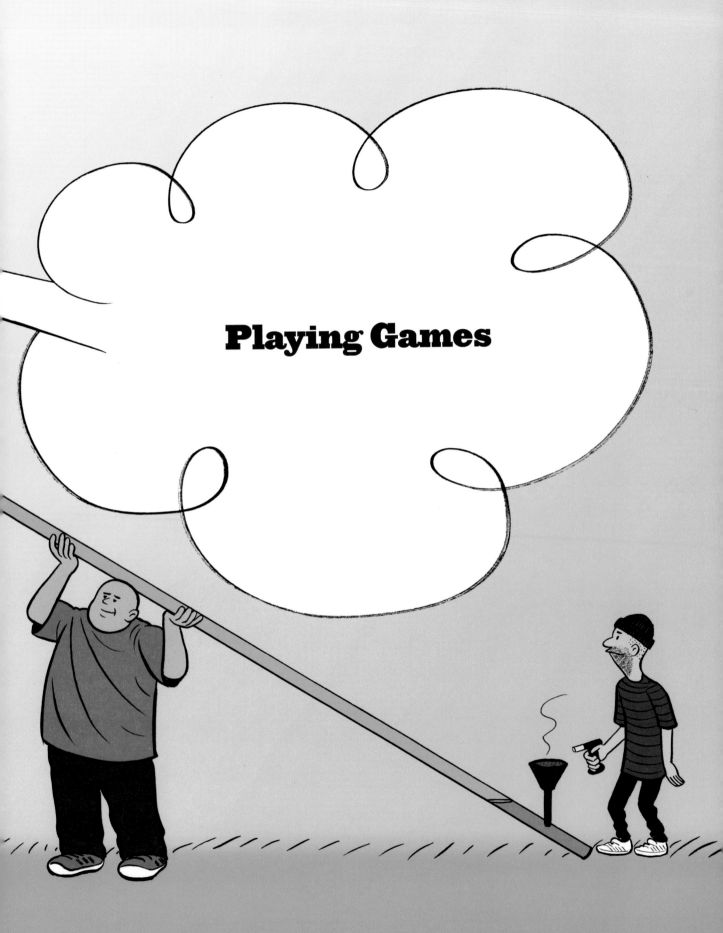

96. COLORING PAGE

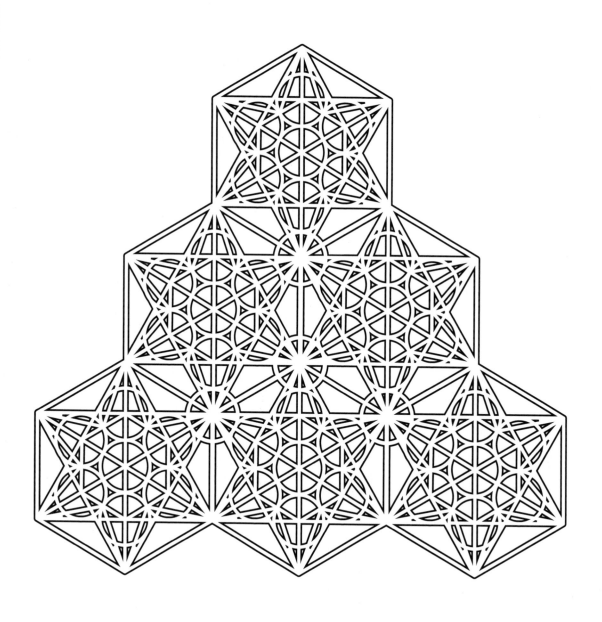

97. FINDING STUFF

ACTION BRONSON IS HAVING A CRAZY DREAM— CAN YOU FIND ALL THE RANDOM SHIT HIDDEN IN IT?

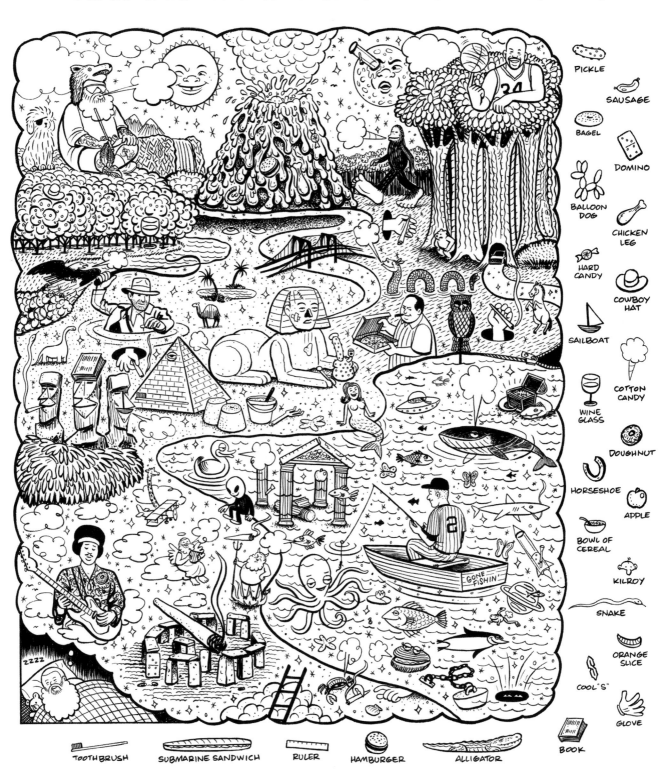

PICKLE
SAUSAGE
BAGEL
DOMINO
BALLOON DOG
CHICKEN LEG
HARD CANDY
COWBOY HAT
SAILBOAT
COTTON CANDY
WINE GLASS
DOUGHNUT
HORSESHOE
APPLE
BOWL OF CEREAL
KILROY
SNAKE
ORANGE SLICE
COOL "S"
GLOVE
BOOK

TOOTHBRUSH · SUBMARINE SANDWICH · RULER · HAMBURGER · ALLIGATOR

98. WORD SEARCH

```
                  B E R Q E U S Y U A
                H O W M Q W W Q W U G R N P
              K O Q D N J I J X A B K K G H B N J
            H L W Y E X N Y G W H E R D R I F W O T
          H N H N J B G L T G K M E M C G S D J E W W
        Y Y H E Q N       F N B H E B       Q K P R O O
      I W L A D Y X       E F Q D P F       C J E D G Y
      G I F O Y W T       R X L R A A       H O S Z J W G
    W G A R B J R K       J O Z K T B       C F C F Y L Q T
    F J Z I Y P G A       S Q B P T L       R X I P N V Q K
  K Y K C F L B T L       Q T G W Y E       N Q J J M G H O T
  M C L L M D D W P       U I U U Z W       Z Q A L O E S W J
  D Y T E M B G T J       E V H N B L       C Y B G N L K Q M
  F C R E D N U H T E T A L O C O H C Q I I Y W X I T Q W J Y
  N R E R E L D U O V W D S T R A N S C E N D E N T A L C U B
  O E I J O D A L E H F N J A R A N E S E C R E A M P U F F T
  I Y N N E P N C H R I S S Y M O L T I S A N T I G S O Q M X
  I P U E R T O R I C A N P O C K E T K N I F E A Z Q K Y J Z
  G N F G D   G I G I K C O C O B L A C K G O A T   D A I R M
  R J N Q I   P H X U E M P A Y T O N O P O P   L P H J B
    W Z Y E   J O E P E S C E P A U E F O Z   N Z U S
    G L L T S                           H D E R G
    Z I F Q O                           R U B Z G
    M L X R G D                         I U S T A M
      T B H D L H J N P J E T R E U F L E A G E M O W
      W N A D D I C T I O N K Y O S Q C D S M O O
      H E Y O D R A V E L U O B A N E S S I K
      M P H H A I R D R E S S E R P Y W I
        O C V B G A N B L U G O J C
        R L Y D L J P T Z B
```

ADDICTION	GOGO	MATSUI
BEEFPATTY	HAIRDRESSER	OMEGAELFUERTE
BLACKGOAT	HELADO	PAYTON
BLICKY	JAPANESECREAMPUFF	PENNY
CHOCOLATETHUNDER	JOEPESCE	POPO
CHRISSYMOLTISANTI	JOEPESCI	PUERTORICANPOCKETKNIFE
COCO	KEMP	SHAQ
EWING	KISSENABOULEVARD	TRANSCENDENTAL
GIGI	LILY	WOK

99. TRIVIA

1. In 1993, who was the inaugural grand champion of the first UFC championship? That was UFC 1, the first-ever event to determine a superior fighter in every fighting style and of martial arts, an eight-man tournament with no rules and no judges.

2. Who has the most World's Strongest Man titles? *Without looking, I am going to guess Žydrūnas Savickas. I was wrong.* It was my second guess. Now I made it easier for you. So now you have to give me the top three people with the most World's Strongest Man titles, and you gotta give me the country where they're from.

3. In the movie *City Slickers II*, what was Billy Crystal going to look for?

4. Give me five more Billy Crystal movies.

5. What is rumored to be buried below Lake Titicaca?

6. What is Tina Turner's favorite color?

7. Who is Alemayehu Esthete?

100. SCRATCH PAPERS

Acknowledgments

I am just happy to be on this earth, or wherever we are, conscious and alert and happy here at this very moment. Right here, right now.

RECIPE INDEX

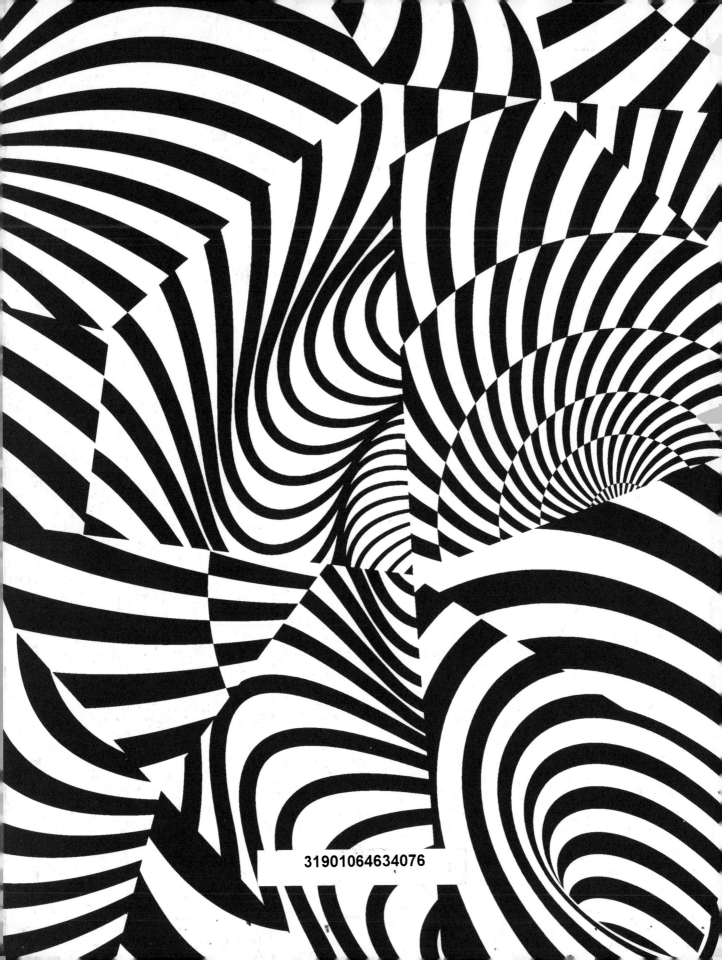